SCHOOL NURSING

To My Mother
Sarah Adeline Slack S.R.N.
With Love and Thanks

School Nursing

**A basic introduction to nursing in
primary and secondary education**

PATRICIA A. SLACK
S.R.N., S.C.M., H.V. Cert., Dip. H. Ed.
Area Nurse (Child Health) Kensington, Chelsea
and Westminster Area Health Authority (Teaching)

BAILLIÈRE TINDALL · LONDON

A BAILLIÈRE TINDALL book published by
Cassell Ltd
35 Red Lion Square, London WC1R 4SG
and at Sydney, Auckland, Toronto, Johannesburg
an affiliate of
Macmillan Publishing Co. Inc.
New York

© 1978 Baillière Tindall
A division of Cassell Ltd

First published 1978

ISBN 0 7020 0672 6

Printed in Great Britain at The Spottiswoode Ballantyne Press
by William Clowes and Sons, Limited, London, Colchester and Beccles

British Library Cataloguing in Publication Data

Slack, Patricia A.
    School nursing.
    1. School children—Health and hygiene
    —Great Britain 2. School nursing—Great
    Britain
    I. Title
    613'.0432   LB3409.G7

ISBN 0-7020-0672-6

Contents

Preface

As a nation we now believe that education for our children is a major priority and in 1907, only a lifetime ago, the school health service was set up to ensure that children were not prevented from achieving their full educational potential through sickness or ill-health. The first school doctors and nurses struggled with problems of malnutrition, physical handicap, infectious diseases and the effects of appalling living conditions experienced by many families.

The psychological and social problems of our present society are reflected in the pattern of ill-health among school children and present a challenge to the personnel of Education, Health and Social Services to work together in the interests of the child. We are also aware that an increasingly large percentage of adult illness is the result of attitudes and health behaviour acquired in childhood. Consequently, education to establish good health habits during these critical years is of prime importance.

Research into school health services has highlighted the benefits of doctors devoting more time to children with complex health and social problems and consequently school nurses have an increasingly important role to play in the identification of sensory defects and in monitoring the physical and mental health of apparently normal children. Additionally, there is continuing responsibility to provide nursing care to handicapped children in ordinary or special schools.

Recently, the health and happiness of children has again been brought to public attention by the publication of *Fit for the Future*, the report of the Committee on Child Health Services headed by Professor Donald Court; this re-emphasized the importance of good health for education and the urgent need to train more doctors and nurses in this area. Their simple definition of school health embodies everything a school nurse needs to aim to be and do.

Educational medicine is the study and practice of child health and paediatrics in relation to the processes of learning. It requires an understanding of child development, the educational environment, the child's response to schooling, the disorders which interfere with a child's capacity to learn, and the special needs of the handicapped. Its practitioners need to work co-operatively with the teachers, psychologists and others who may be involved with the child and to understand the influences of family and social environment.

In this book I have set out to equip the nurse with a basis from which to start planning and organizing her work in school. I assume that some knowledge of child development and children's illnesses has been acquired during basic training and I try to show her how this knowledge may be applied and extended for use in schools.

The bibliography provides suggestions for further reading and I hope that many of the children's books will find their way into more school libraries and medical rooms; I hope too that these books will be read by nurses themselves. The much-fingered, much-read tattered children's book can teach the adult a lot about the interests and view-point of the child as well as giving nurses and teachers another dimension to explore in their conversations with children. Books written for children particularly in recent years often present the predicaments of children in a manner much more striking than is usual in adult reference books.

Recently, I had a spontaneous conversation with a nine-year-old in the children's library who suggested I read *The Trouble with Donovan Croft* (see p. 100). 'That's a real good story', she said. 'Why?' I asked. 'Dunno,' she said, 'he's a bit like a kid we had to stay with us'; so I read about Donovan and his reaction to a situation experienced by many West Indian children in inner cities.

Books about visits to doctors, dentists or nurses and books which describe examinations or immunizations can be used to engender a positive attitude in children so that they understand what is going to happen and why. Story books concerning handicapped children or social and marital situations can lead parents and other children to a better understanding of an unhappy child and may be encouraging for the child himself. However, if they are used as a teaching aid they do need to be examined by the nurse and teacher, and in some circumstances by the doctor or child psychiatrist, because some of the stories dealing with subjects such as mental handicap, autism or difficult relationships might not be in the best interests of a child.

The discussion topics at the end of each chapter, while designed primarily to recapitulate and illustrate the practical application of the chapter, have much wider implications which I hope will lead the nurse to further exploration and interest in the subject.

School nursing is a field wide open for development and research and it needs nurses of talent and ability to explore its full potential. I hope that some will be encouraged by the very existence of this book and that children everywhere will benefit from their efforts.

I should like to thank everyone who contributed to my efforts. The following helped in my search for information: Mrs Allen, School Matron, Hampshire School Matrons Association; Mr John Cleary, Area Dental Officer; Dr Bethan Davies, Consultant Audiologist; Miss Pam Hay, Council for Education and Training of Health Visitors; Miss Fox, Children's Librarian; Mr Hopkins, P. C. Worth Ltd; Miss Kate Jones, Librarian, Royal Society of Health; Dr Sparks and Sister Russell, Rugby School; the Nursing and Education staff in ILEA, Kent and Hampshire Schools.

Those who gave up their time to read and comment on various sections of the script included: Mr Ray Amer, Health Education Officer; Miss Stella Earl, Nursing Officer, DHSS; Mrs Hill, School Sister; Dr Anne Jepson, Area Specialist in Community Medicine (Child Health); Miss Edna Llewellyn, Principal Lecturer in Health Studies; Mrs Mules, Health Visitor; Mrs O'Brien, School Sister; Mrs Radwanski, Health and Safety Executive; Miss Simms, Peripatetic Teacher for the Partially-sighted; Mrs M. Thornton and Miss Sara Lomas, Disabled Living Foundation; Mr Don Venvell, Assistant Education Officer; Miss Lynn Weekes, Optical Information Council; Dr Harry Zeitlin, Consultant Child Psychiatrist; the staff of Cheyne Centre.

I should also like to thank everyone who supplied visual material to illustrate the text, including Ann Arvanitakis RIBA who designed the plan of the medical accommodation and her daughter Zanthe, and Marie, Michael and Candide Bott who posed for photographs and Mr Robert McCrum, photographer; and last but by no means least the staff of Baillière Tindall, and Miss Sumi Tikaram who gave up so many precious evenings to type the script so meticulously.

February, 1978   PATRICIA A. SLACK

1

The Education Service

A nurse who ceases to work in hospital and begins to work in a school leaves a rarified atmosphere where diagnosis of illness and methods of treatment and care are the major all-absorbing interest. She now chooses to practise and apply the skills she has acquired in a totally different setting dominated by theories of educational philosophy and practice. Just as a patient who has experienced the health service as a consumer cannot assume to have any knowledge of medicine, a nurse cannot assume to know about education through having experienced school. Therefore, if she is to be accepted as a valuable staff member and practise her profession to full advantage she must begin by understanding the rudiments of the system and the function of the staff in the schools to which she is attached.

The history of education dates back beyond the ancient Greek philosophers, Plato and Aristotle, and since then to the present day there has been a diversity of speculations and theories relating to the purpose of education and what it is expected to achieve as well as the best methods of teaching. Today in England, education is a major political issue which can be argued from any number of viewpoints on which it would be inappropriate to comment here.

Our British education system dates back to the establishment of the church and remained largely its province until the dissolution of the monasteries. Indeed, some of our existing public schools can trace their origins back beyond the establishment of the universities of Oxford and Cambridge in the twelfth or thirteenth century to the early 'grammar' schools set up to teach Latin and the classics.

Following the reign of Henry VIII, the remaining schools were supported and new ones established by rich benefactors, including the church, and education flourished even to the extent of providing many free places and also free schools out of public money. The Industrial Revolution, however, sent children into the mines and factories as cheap labour and large numbers of schools were closed. Britain was, nevertheless, struggling to become an industrial power and needed educated people to achieve this; consequently, a group of leading figures pressed for a national system of elementary education and this was proposed and rejected by Parliament in 1807. In the meantime, voluntary organizations supported by the church set out with some success to establish this aim and in 1833 they received a government grant which became an annual arrangement, administered by the committee of the Privy Council on Education, the forerunner of the present Department of Education and Science (DES), which distinguished itself by increasing the subjects taught, introducing training for teachers and establishing Her Majesty's Inspectorate to advise. Finally in 1870 the Elementary Education Act struggled through Parliament making provision for the election of school boards to set up schools where there was no voluntary provision, and to enforce attendance if they so wished.

Meanwhile, movement was also starting in secondary education and vocational courses in technical colleges and at evening classes were also developing. Special education for handicapped children was gaining recognition since the establishment of the first schools for the deaf (1760) and blind (1791), and in 1899 a National Board of Education was set up to supervise elementary, secondary and vocational education and to make provision for the defective and epileptic child (the deaf and blind having had statutory provision made in 1893). This was followed by the Education Act (1902) which made provision for additional financial support from local rates. School boards were abolished and county and county boroughs became local education authorities with a duty to provide elementary education up to the age of 14 years (or 13 in some cases) and permissive powers to provide financial aid to other areas of education. The result for secondary education was patchy provision depending on the priorities of the local authority; this was further complicated by the 1907 regulations which required a proportion of free places to be set aside in maintained or 'aided' schools for pupils paid for by the local education authority; consequently, as secondary education began at 11 years and places were few, the selection became highly competitive.

Children remaining in the elementary system had no equivalent secondary courses until the 1918 Education Act which imposed a duty on local authorities to provide suitable courses for older abler elementary children as well as raising the leaving age to 14 years for all children, irrespective of circumstances. The resulting courses received the seal of approval with the 'Haddow' Report (1926)[1] which recommended that junior or primary education end at 11 years and senior or secondary education to provide until school leaving and be known as 'modern'. Junior technical colleges which had developed were recognized as a suitable part of the secondary provision only in 1938.

During the Second World War it became clear that further reforms were needed. This led to the 1944 Education Act[2] which remains the basis of our present system. The most important proposals in context of school nursing in primary and secondary schools are summarized very briefly as follows.

Section 1 A Minister and Ministry of Education was established (became the Secretary of State for Education and Science and the Department of Education and Science in 1964).

Section 6 and schedule 1 Local authorities of county and county boroughs became local education authorities (under the 1963 Local Government Act the Greater London Council became the Inner London Education Authority, acting on behalf of the twelve inner London boroughs; the outer London boroughs became separate education authorities; the 1972 Local Government Act provided a reorganized structure outside Greater London and came into force in 1974, creating 45 new counties, 39 of which are responsible for education). County councils might, for administrative purposes, create divisions to exercise specified functions in relation to primary and secondary education. Each local education authority were to appoint an education committee or joint education committees between two or more local education authorities. The majority of the committee were to be members of the authority but to include persons with experience in education and also persons acquainted with education conditions prevailing in the area.

Sections 7, 8, 9 and 15 Public education was organized in three stages—primary, secondary and further education—with the local education authority having a duty 'to contribute towards the spiritual, moral, mental and physical development of the community by ensuring that sufficient education throughout those stages shall be available to meet the needs of the population of their area'. They should also give particular attention to:

a. providing primary and secondary education in separate buildings, except in the case of special schools;
b. providing nursery schools and classes for children under five years;
c. provision of special educational treatment for children with mental or physical disabilities (these were to be categorized and special schools provided);
d. provision of boarding accommodation as thought desirable in the interests of the child.

Schools established by the education authority were to be known as county schools and those established by others to be known as voluntary. However, voluntary schools might be: controlled (all expenses paid by local education authority, property remains in possession of voluntary organization); aided (local education authority pays running cost, voluntary organization pays part of capital costs and retains building); special agreement (local education authority grants 50 to 75% of building cost).

Sections 17 to 21 All schools should have a board of managers (primary level) or governors (secondary level). The former to be not less than six persons and the latter number to be determined by the local education authority. In county schools they would be appointed by the authority and in voluntary controlled schools one-third would be appointed by the voluntary body and two-thirds in the case of aided and special agreement schools. Two or more schools could be grouped under one board. (Functions of boards of managers and governors reviewed by the Taylor Committee and published in September, 1977.)

Sections 33 and 34 The local education authority had a duty to discover children requiring special educational treatment. In order to do this they would seek the advice of a medical officer who would examine the child to determine the nature of their disability and advise the authority and the parents accordingly.

Sections 36 to 40 It would be a duty of parents to see that their child received suitable education either in the school or elsewhere between the ages of 5 and 15 years, the school leaving age at a later date to be raised to 16 years (achieved 1973). Parents whose children did not attend school and who could not satisfy the authority that suitable alternative provision was made or that the child was absent for sickness, observance of religion, without transport, or of no fixed abode, would be served with a 'School Attendance Order' and be liable to conviction. To secure attendance, the juvenile court could, if necessary, place an order to have the child taken into care of the local authority.

The local education authority had a duty to provide all the following ancillary services:

Sections 48 Regular medical inspection and free treatment (repealed by the NHS Reorganization 1973) to all children and to encourage the pupils to take advantage of these facilities.

Sections 49 Milk, meals and other refreshments.

Section 53 Facilities for recreation and social and physical training. This may include establishing or helping to maintain camps, holiday classes, playing-fields, play centres, playgrounds, gymnasiums and swimming baths.

Section 54 To make arrangements for cleansing verminous children and their clothing and to authorize a medical officer to arrange examinations of pupils to determine the necessity for this. The medical officer may, if necessary, exclude the child from school and if repeated infestation occurs, and neglect can be proved, the parent or pupil may be prosecuted.

Section 59 Give written notice to a parent of a child who has reached the age of two and is thought to be mentally defective; to submit the child for medical examination by a doctor of the authority. The time and place to be specified and the parent entitled to be present. The purpose of this to determine whether the child was capable of receiving education in school. Any child attending a maintained or special school requiring supervision on leaving school because of such a disability, the local authority and the parent to be notified of this.

(Repealed in 1970 when Education (Handicapped Children) Act made provision for their education.)

The local education authority were also empowered to secure the following:

Section 50 Boarding facilities if necessary.

Section 51 Clothing if inadequate and if interfering with the child's education (repealed by 1948 Education (Miscellaneous Provisions) Act).

Section 55 Transport facilities to enable children to attend school. (At present if under 8 years and 2 miles from school and over 8 years and 3 miles. from school; local education authorities may either pay fares on public transport or provide their own.)

Section 56 Alternative facilities for child to be educated other than in school.

Sections 58 to 60 Prohibit an employer from continuing to employ a child if the duties interfered with health or education.

Sections 70 and 78 All independent schools (any school not maintained or supported by the local education authority which provides full-time education for five or more pupils) to be registered by an officer appointed by the Minister. Local education authorities were empowered to provide medical inspection and treatment, milk, meals and other refreshments, together with clothing, if necessary, providing the expense does not exceed the cost if the pupil attended a maintained school.

Section 77 The Minister (Secretary of State for Education and Science) has a duty to cause inspections of every educational establishment by inspectors to be appointed by Her Majesty (HMIs). Local education authorities could also appoint inspectors to inspect the authority's maintained schools.

Section 80 Every school to keep a register of pupils.

Since 1944 the important developments to consider here have occurred in the schools themselves and within the first two of the following stages of education:

1. Primary 2 to 11 years (may finish any time between $10\frac{1}{2}$ and 12th birthday).
2. Secondary 11 to 18 years (compulsory until 16 years). Since 1964 development of middle schools designated either primary or secondary for below $10\frac{1}{2}$ to above 12 years; usually 8 to 12 or 9 to 13 years.
3. University and further education—adults.

Primary Education

Primary education may be divided into the following phases:

Nursery	2–5 years.
Infant	5–7 + years.
Junior	7+–11+ years.

Nursery education provides ideal opportunities for children to start socializing and to learn and experience the world through play and it is a particularly valuable experience for children from homes where there is little or no stimulation to either the child's speech and language or physical and mental development. Indeed, the Plowden Report[3] which was an important influence on primary education went to some length to emphasize the need for expansion of nursery education and positive discrimination for socially deprived areas. Since 1968 urban aid grants have been available to provide nursery schools and classes together with day nurseries and children's homes in areas where there is overcrowding or where more than 6% of the population are immigrants. Pressures from parents in other areas led to the rapid development of the pre-school playgroups movement to fill the gap, and in 1972 a government white paper entitled 'Education—A Framework for Expansion'[4] promised massive increases in nursery education although the subsequent economic decline has hampered developments.

At five years compulsory schooling begins and children enter the infants school the first year of which is known as the 'reception' class. Activities here are largely a gradual extension of nursery education to a more structured though informal pattern and children may be taught in groups of either similar or various ages (family grouping). The infant's school may be housed in a separate building with a separate head teacher from the junior school, or they may be combined in one building with a single head responsible for both groups.

The junior school aims to teach not only basic literacy and numeracy but also encourages children to explore a wide variety of interests and subjects.

Secondary Education

Towards the end of primary education and the beginning of secondary education, education authorities must endeavour to discover what sort of secondary education is most suited to each child. Various methods of testing children have been used, the most well-known being the 11+ examination which has now been replaced by long-term methods of assessment.

Secondary school provision available since 1944 has been of three types—grammar, technical and secondary modern.

The *grammar school* was the most academic, educating children to take the general certificate of education (GCE), ordinary and advanced level, usually with a view to university or higher education.

The *secondary technical school*, although conceived as the equivalent of the grammar school, but with a bias towards technology, never, in fact, became very popular and there have been few.

The *secondary modern schools* replaced the senior elementary school and were encouraged to develop courses in the best interests of individual pupils. A wide range of vocational courses began to be provided; indeed, some schools also entered children for the GCE and in 1965 the certificate of secondary education

(CSE) was introduced, the highest grade of which is equivalent to GCE ordinary level pass.

This tripartite system was meant to be flexible and to achieve this further, bilateral schools (combinations of any two of the above three) or the more widespread comprehensive schools (combinations of all three for secondary ages in an area) grew up, particularly since 1965. The 1976 Education Act states that this type of education can only be provided in schools where there is no selection by ability or aptitude. Comprehensive schools may be organized in a variety of ways:

1. 'All through' (11 to 18 years).
2. Junior and senior comprehensive (all transfer from one to the other at 13 or 14 years).
3. Junior and senior comprehensive (some transfer to senior at 13 or 14 years for further education; rest remain at junior level until school-leaving).
4. Junior and two senior comprehensive (all transfer at 13 or 14 to either senior for children up to 16 years, or senior for children to remain longer).
5. Comprehensive (11 to 16 years) followed by optional sixth-form college.
6. Comprehensive middle school 8–9 to 12–13 years (transfer to comprehensive 12–13 to 18 years).

The numbers of children per building will vary but where numbers are large (up to 2000 children), particular care is needed in providing a satisfactory system of administration and 'pastoral' care (see p. 96) so that children are not overwhelmed by sheer size and numbers.

Special Education

The local authority must provide education for all children and the system of assessment for special education, together with the facilities at present available, is described in Chapter 8. At the time of writing, the question of special education is being examined by a government committee under the chairmanship of Mrs Mary Warnock.

Independent Schools

At present there are about 2200 independent schools in the country. Preparatory school usually starts at eight years and finishes between 12 and 14 years when an examination, known as Common Entrance, is taken to gain admission to a secondary independent school. These are often 'public' schools which is the term usually applied to those establishments which are members of the Head Masters Conference, the Governing Bodies Association or the Governing Bodies of Girls Schools Association. All independent schools have to be registered with the Department of Education and submit to regular inspection. Some schools also apply to be 'recognized as efficient' which involves more rigorous inspection. However, it should not be assumed that a school which does not carry this recognition is of a low-standard because application is purely voluntary. Indeed, because of recent financial restraint, this extra inspection may have to be dropped. The Department of Education and Science List No. 70 gives details, including fees and size of all 'recognized efficient schools'. A comprehensive account of each individual school, its educational aims and staffing arrangements is given in 'The Public and Preparatory School Year Book' which is published yearly and is available from the local reference library.

Further Education

This applies to all types of adult education including universities, polytechnics, colleges of further education and adult institutes.

School Staff

It is important to understand something of the function and background of school staff with whom there may be contact. These may be divided into two groups: those who work in the school daily and those who visit for specific purposes from time to time.

Permanent staff *Teachers* These form the major and most influential part of the service, the head teacher having considerable influence and autonomy within his or her school. Primary teachers usually undertake the teaching of all subjects to their class while at secondary level it is usual to specialize in one or two subjects.

Recognized teaching qualifications are necessary for anyone undertaking the teaching of children except where speakers are invited as experts on their particular subject, or in special circumstances where there is a shortage of trained teachers for a particular subject. Qualifications may be a university degree followed by a one-year teacher-training or a three-year course at a college of education (before 1960, a two-year course was considered sufficient). Some colleges also run four-year courses for teachers wishing to gain a batchelor of education degree. The minimum educational requirements for entry to teacher-training colleges are five GCE 'O' levels or three GCE 'O' levels, together with one 'A' level, or three 'A' levels with evidence of having studied other subjects. Exceptions are teachers of art who follow a one-year course, the entry requirement being a professional qualification as an artist or craftsman.

Those qualified in other countries wishing to take up employment here must apply for recognition. Since 1965 special courses have been set up to actively encourage teachers qualified in New Commonwealth countries to take up teaching here, particularly in schools with large numbers of children whose parents are immigrants.

Teachers working in special schools or with special classes for vision or hearing defect require an additional qualification which is usually taken following two years teaching experience in ordinary school. Training is not obligatory for those coping with other handicaps although it is increasingly recognized as necessary.

There are also many refresher and short courses run by the DES, institutes of education or professional organizations. Additionally, local authorities usually provide a variety of short in-service courses often at teachers' centres set up for this purpose. Sometimes these are inter-disciplinary and open to health service staff.

The school secretary and the caretaker There is generally one school secretary in a primary school and possibly several in a large school to assist the head teacher and staff with secretarial work and the general clerical administration. They usually know the parents and have a good knowledge of the movements of children and teachers. It is extremely important for a nurse to develop a good relationship with the secretarial staff as it is from here that up-to-date lists of new entrants, pupils and teachers, as well as time-tables and programmes, will be issued. A co-operative secretary will usually act as a 'post-box' for messages and may give considerable assistance in contacting parents.

The caretaker is responsible for security and general up-keep, including the cleaning arrangements, repairs, and supplies, and often lives on the premises. He is particularly important in the effect he may have on accident prevention and in arranging access to the school outside school hours when it may be useful to complete clerical work, for example.

School helpers School helpers are lay members of staff employed to help teachers generally. Their duties may include class-room activities and the preparation of teaching materials, supervision of play and meals and escort duties within and outside the school. They may assist at medical and nursing examinations by fetching the children to and from class and frequently they are given responsibility for first-aid in which case it is necessary to ensure that they are made aware of any special problems a child may have.

Handicapped children may need special assistance with using the lavatory and moving around the school. Special schools usually employ lay helpers known as care assistants for this purpose.

Staff responsible for cooking, serving and washing up after meals may be responsible to the head teacher or to the school meals organizer employed by the local education authority to make arrangements for adequate nutritious meals to be served and to maintain high standards of hygiene.

Visiting staff *School inspectors* Her Majesty's Inspectors (HMIs) from the DES may visit independent or maintained schools to assess the education standard, the facilities available and the school buildings. Inspections of maintained schools may also be made by the local education authority inspectors who act as an important link presenting the difficulties and needs of individual schools to the authority.

Specialist and advisory teachers Specialist and advisory teachers may be employed in the school to give assistance to children with special needs as, for example, slow readers in need of remedial teaching. Alternatively, they may be peripatetic and visit the school either to provide special help for a child or advise the class teacher about the management of a problem such as a partially-sighted child in an ordinary school.

Educational psychologists Members of the school psychological service, which exists to help teachers with children who have persistent learning difficulties, spend a good deal of time interviewing such children and carrying out psychological tests. Following these tests they will advise the teacher and may help with planning suitable curricula for these children. Learning difficulties may arise from physical or emotional problems and for this reason it is essential that the educational psychologist works closely with the school doctor and the child psychiatrist and he is usually attached to the local child guidance or hospital child psychiatric team. It should be explained here that child guidance was a service provided by local education authorities to deal with children having emotional and behaviour problems. The team consisted of a consultant child psychiatrist, educational psychologist, psychiatric social worker and possibly a psychotherapist. Since 1974 the various members of these teams are employed and responsible to their respective authorities: doctors to the NHS, social workers to Social Services and educationalists to the education authority. The service continues to be provided and is likely to extend to children below school entry, attending child health clinics, day nurseries or nursery classes.

The numbers of educational psychologists and the range of help they are able to offer varies considerably throughout the country, depending on the numbers employed to meet the need. Some voluntary organizations such as the Spastics Society also employ educational psychologists to offer a national service to the children they are concerned with.

The educational psychologist usually has a university degree in psychology, followed by postgraduate training in educational psychology together with three years or more experience in teaching.

Education welfare officer Welfare officers are members of the education welfare service which grew out of the need to enforce school attendance where children were frequently absent from school. School attendance officers were appointed to serve notices on parents and ultimately to take them to court. Inevitably, the reasons for the children staying at home were not entirely straightforward. Children were often kept at home because they had neither suitable clothing nor shoes or because parents could not afford transport or school meals; some children were also illegally employed. The 1944 Act, as we have seen, placed this responsibility firmly with education authorities and later the Plowden

Report[3] emphasized the need to help families whose difficulties adversely affected a child's school performance. Consequently, in most authorities these duties are carried out by the education welfare service.

The service is still growing and the range of responsibilities undertaken by individual authorities varies considerably. Some authorities still see the work as concerned primarily with court proceedings for truancy while others, in consultation with social services, have extended the role to include even the supervision of children under care orders. There is, therefore, a gradual extension of the work to overlap with that of social services and it is often difficult to determine in whose province a particular problem may fall. Indeed, many are of the opinion that the two services will eventually be merged. The 1968 Seebohm Report on Social Services[5] did in fact recommend this and a few authorities adopted the suggestion. However, it did not seem to be very successful and they have reverted to the previous arrangements.

Before 1964, education welfare officers had no recognized qualification nor indeed was one available to them until the local government training board set up a day-release course leading to a certificate in Education Welfare. However, by 1971 only 8.5% of education welfare officers held this qualification[6]. Since then some authorities, taking heed of the Report of the Local Government Training Board, have seconded staff for professional social work courses and appointed training officers to set up in-service training programmes for existing staff.

The situation in London is somewhat complicated by the fact that there are a large number of voluntary workers known as care committee workers who are part of the education welfare service. This has a long-standing history in London and at one time the entire provision of shoes, clothing and general social support was in their hands. Most of them are very experienced, highly efficient and very valuable assets to the schools, particularly as they live and work in the area and provide stability whereas salaried employees tend to be somewhat transient.

Careers officer Careers officers are employed by the local education authority to help children and parents plan a future career. They work closely with youth employment officers and disablement resettlement officers in finding suitable employment and training for both normal and handicapped children. The careers officer has responsibility for seeing every child and his parents or guardian to discuss the child's future, usually between 13 and 16 years of age. Consideration must be given to the child's ability and attainment, his temperament and any special aptitudes or interests he may have. His home circumstances and the amount of support he can hope to have from his parents are important guidelines as well as his general health and physique. Personal discussion is usually backed up by talks to groups of children and general information on careers available. Good communication between school health personnel and careers officers is essential, particularly where a child is handicapped. Forms for this purpose are designed to be used at the school-leaving medical: form Y9 to be used for ordinary children, and Y10 for the handicapped. Forms, however, must not take the place of personal communication which is essential in certain circumstances.

Careers officers are usually recruited from a variety of backgrounds, the criteria being practical broadly-based work experience of at least two years. This is followed by a one-year course at a polytechnic or university.

Youth officer As we have seen under the 1944 Act, local education authorities have responsibility to see that there are suitable leisure activities for adolescents living in their area and youth officers are employed to develop these. They may encourage adolescents to join activities run by any of the many voluntary organizations such as the scout and guide movement, St John's Ambulance Brigade or the Youth Hostels Organization. They may also establish youth centres, often in school premises, and recruit instructors for games, art, drama and whatever is of interest to the individual group. They have an increasingly important role to play in establishing patterns of social and leisure activities particularly in culturally deprived areas with a lack of outlet for adolescent energies and they provide good back-up for the pastoral care and welfare services in the school.

Parents and the community Children spend a large part of their days and their lives in school and it is desirable for the school, the child and the parents that there should be good communications and that parents should be involved. The degree of involvement will vary, depending on the school staff and the interest or otherwise of parents. In some schools communication may be limited to formal or informal individual interviews and in others there may be flourishing parent–teacher association meetings where items of mutual concern may be discussed. These meetings may be a useful contact for the school health team and the possibilites can be discussed with the head teacher. Boards of governors and managers may include a parent representative, often elected by the parents themselves.

Finally, the school is a focus in a community and as such may be a social centre and point of contact of considerable significance and importance to individual families and the local community. Many schools encourage health education, social studies and community involvement as part of the curricula and children and adolescents will often provide a valuable social service to the elderly, needy or lonely in the vicinity. This may be mutual if adults are encouraged to take an active part in helping with school outings, plays, entertainments and money-raising activities.

REFERENCES

1. The Haddow Report (1926) *The Education of the Adolescent.* London: Board of Education, HMSO.

2. The Education Act (1944) London: HMSO.
3. The Plowden Report (1967) *Children and Their Primary Schools—A Report of the Central Advisory Council for Education (England)*. London: HMSO.
4. DES Cmnd 5174 *Education: A Framework for Expansion*. London: HMSO.
5. Seebohm Report (1968) *Report of the Committee on Local Authority and Allied Personal Social Services*. London: HMSO, Cmnd 3703.
6. The Ralphs Report (1972) *The Role and Training of Education Welfare Officers: Summary of Report of the Working Party*. London: Local Government Training Board, HMSO.

FURTHER READING

Bourne, R. (1975) *Choosing a School*, Cambridge: Advisory Centre for Education.
Clarke, J. J. (1969) *Outline of Local Government of the United Kingdom*, 20th ed. London: Pitman.
Central Office of Information (1974) *Education in Britain Pamphlet 7, 6th ed.* London: HMSO.
Davies, L. (1976) Education Welfare Surveyed. *Community Care*, 98, pp 16–17.
Dent, H. C. (1971) *The Education System of England and Wales*, 5th ed. London: Unibooks.
DES (1973) *Careers Education in Secondary Schools: Education Survey 18*. London: HMSO.
Stone, J. & Taylor, F. (1976) *The Parents School Book*. London: Pelican.
The Summerfield Report (1968) *Psychologists in Educational Services*. London: HMSO.
Taylor Report (1977) *A New Partnership for our Schools*. London: HMSO.

USEFUL ADDRESSES AND INFORMATION

Advisory Centre for Education
32 Trumpington Street
Cambridge.
Tel: 0223 (Cambridge) 51456.

Provides an advisory service on all aspects of education, primarily for parents. Produces a number of publications including a monthly magazine 'Where' which frequently carries articles about school health.

Her Majesty's Stationery Office
(Nearest local address obtainable from telephone directory.)

Publishes free of charge a list of all Department of Education and Science publications which are still in print. This is up-dated every six months and is a useful source of information available.

Discussion Topics

1. During the annual nursing survey you notice that one family of children have badly fitting shoes which are affecting their feet. You already know that there is considerable financial difficulty in the family. Who would be the most appropriate person in the education service to discuss this with?

2. There is a parent–teacher association in the school. Do you think there are occasions when it might be appropriate to attend and how would you arrange this?

3. A 12-year-old boy has suddenly changed his behaviour pattern and becomes very disruptive. He has been prescribed a course of drugs from the chest clinic but has refused to take them and letters to his mother have produced no response. You make a home visit and the mother breaks down and tells you that she is having severe marital problems. Which members of the education service might provide assistance and support to (a) the mother, and (b) the child?

4. Consider whether you feel boards of managers or governors have a role to play in promoting the school health service and what your relationship with them might be.

5. You are appointed to work in a school which has a history of poor relationships with the school health service. Because of the unpleasant atmosphere and the lack of co-operation or recognition given to the work of the school nurse, your two predecessors stayed only a short time. Consider ways in which you might set about achieving recognition and co-operation from the school staff.

6. You are leaving the school to take up another post and you are told that the new school nurse will start a week before you leave so that there is a 'hand-over' period. Consider how she might be satisfactorily introduced to the education personnel and service in the school.

2
The School Health Service

The development of a school health service is closely bound up with the development of a public health service in Britain. The industrial revolution, with the rapid growth of towns, over-crowding and insanitary conditions, created a climate in which disease and illness were rife. Outbreaks of cholera in the 1830s were followed by efforts to improve conditions and in 1848 the first Public Health Act was passed. Medical officers of health began to be appointed to take positive health measures and safeguard the health of the community. By the turn of the century their responsibilities included clean water supply, sewage disposal, sanitation of buildings, removal of nuisances, inspection of food, sanitary burial and notification of infectious diseases.

Meanwhile, some school boards were starting to appoint school doctors to examine the children and following the 1904 Report of the Interdepartmental Committee on Physical Deterioration, which approved the practice, the 1907 Education Act made it a duty of local education authorites to provide medical inspections for children attending public elementary schools (see Fig. 1). This was to be carried out in conjunction with other public health activities under the supervision of the medical officer of health. In 1918 it became an additional duty to provide medical treatment in elementary schools and inspection in secondary schools (treatment was permissive). During these early years the service was in the main curative and, very important, free. Alongside this, developments were progressing for the pre-school child and health visitors were being appointed to visit young children and families in their homes. Both health visiting and school nursing remained the responsibility of local health authorities under the supervision of the medical officer of health until 1974 when the 1973 NHS Reorganization Act came into force.

We have seen from the previous chapter that the 1944 Education Act placed firm responsibility with education authorities to seek the advice of a medical officer in discovering children requiring special education or who were mentally defective, to provide regular medical inspection and free treatment and cleansing of verminous pupils. These have remained the basis of the functions of the school health service, the nurses' duties being mainly in connection with servicing the medical inspections and in carrying out treatments and cleansing.

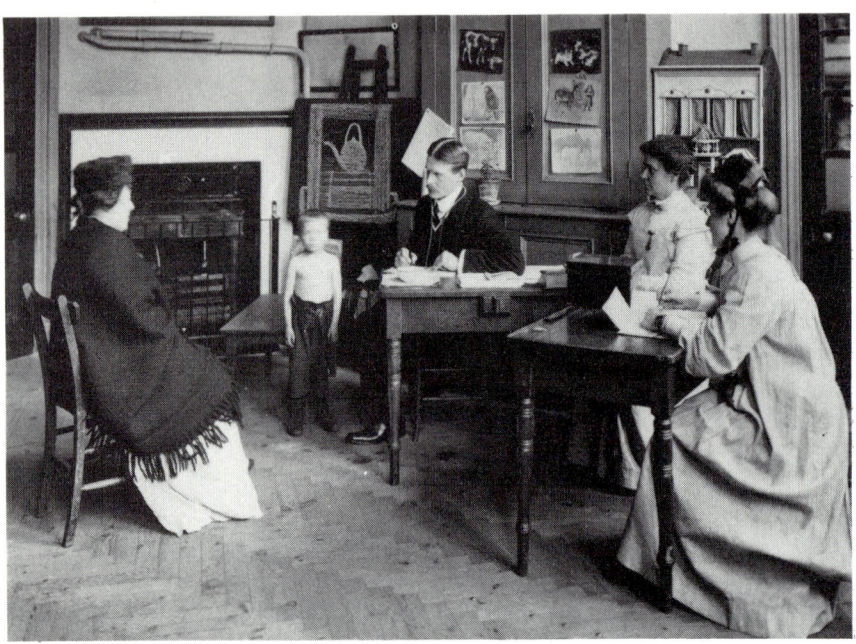

Fig. 1. Medical inspection, Holland Street School, 1903. (GLC Photographic Library)

The 1945 School Health Regulations recommended that all school nurses should be qualified health visitors, emphasizing the broad sense of the role of school nurse envisaged by the authorities. However, for reasons not entirely clear, but possibly connected with the 1959 School Health Regulations, which accepted nurses without health visiting qualifications as school nurses, the role has often been given a restricted interpretation. The belief that school nurses are only capable of examining heads for lice ('Nitty Nora') extends to many teachers as well as pupils and has given little scope for school nurses to fully use their skills.

The 1946 NHS Act made hospital and specialist advice free and gradually the curative role of the school doctor passed to general practitioners and hospital services although the nurse continued to combine her preventive and curative activities.

Many of the independent schools had medical services long before a statutory school health service was created. The 1944 Education Act did however give local education authorities the power to provide medical inspections and treatment for pupils in independent schools. Little has ever come of this and most independent schools contract with independent doctors and nurses although services such as immunization and vaccination or advice on cleansing may sometimes be requested from the statutory school health service. Under the NHS Act 1973 the power to provide services to independent schools passed to the NHS and arrangements may be made with area health authorities.

Section 3 of the 1973 Act also made medical and dental inspection and treatment in maintained schools a function of the NHS and for these purposes health personnel, including doctors, dentists, nurses, speech therapists and others should be made available to support the service. Responsibilities to arrange medical examinations for children needing special educational treatment, making accommodation available and encouraging pupils to take advantage of the service remain with local education authorities.

The aim of the 1973 NHS Act was to combine the segregated health services previously functioning under local health authorities, regional hospital boards, hospital management committees and executive councils. Consequently, the school health service should now be part of an integrated child health service functioning within a district. The national structure under which this is provided is outlined in Fig. 2.

The area specialist in community medicine (child health) and the area nurse (child health) (Fig. 2) are directly responsible for the school health service together with advising on the provision of an integrated child health service; the area dental officer is responsible for the school dental service. The area nurse (child health) works with the district nursing officers in providing the nursing service and information comes through the nurses district management structure.

Section 10 of the 1973 NHS Reorganization Act requires health authorities and local authorities to co-operate together and, to achieve this, machinery for discussing future planning and sharing of resources has been set up between education, health and social services. This is known as the joint consultative committee and is illustrated in Fig. 3. The committee makes decisions on papers presented to them by working groups of officers representing each service.

The area nurse (child health) is normally the officer to represent school nursing on joint consultative committee working groups. Therefore, it it very important that any difficulties arising in schools between health, education and social services interests should be made known to her so that she can fully represent the nurses' point of view. Where she is not informed or aware of

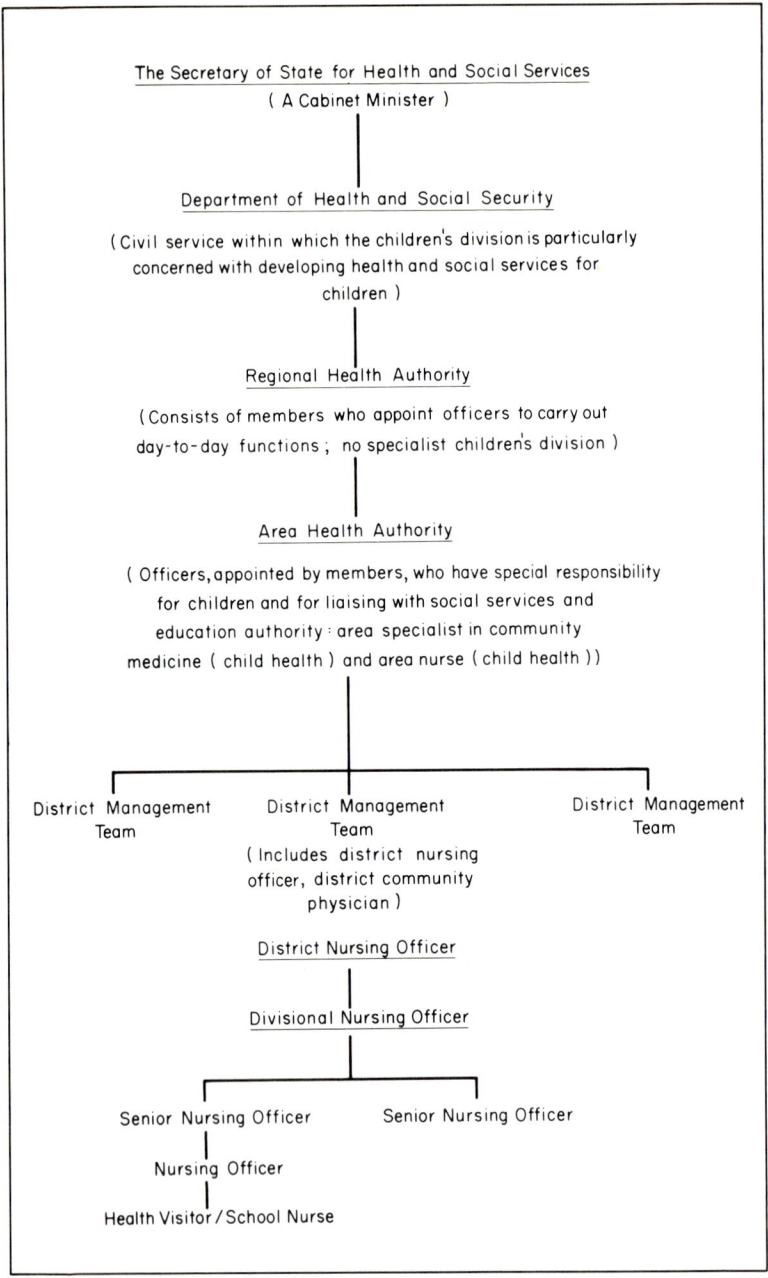

Fig. 2.   The position of school nursing in the structure of the NHS.

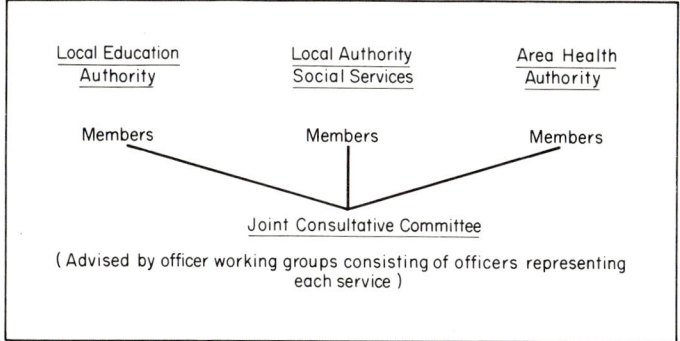

Fig. 3. The joint consultative committee.

problems the nurse and the service may suffer. Additionally, there may be health care planning teams examining services for children at district level and a member of the senior nursing staff will include school nursing in her representation.

This structure may seem complicated and out of the province of the school nurse. However, its very existence is only valuable if it facilitates joint projects within the schools for local day to day working and benefit to the children. Opportunities for co-operation abound and there are many examples of education, health and social services working together for the benefit of the local community and education of the children in school. One example is a primary school attended by many children who in their pre-school years had been cared for by numerous child-minders. The headmistress, worried about the resulting adverse effects on the children's learning, began to explore the situation with the social worker and health visitor. This school now runs a flourishing child-minders' club with attached crèche for their small charges. The adult education institute contributes by arranging a suitable education input on child development and this is backed up by a toy library run by the school and providing suitable play material for the child-minders to borrow.

Another example was the discovery that a number of children excluded from school because of illness were left alone at home all day while their mothers were at work. These were in the main single-parent families where the mother's continuing full-time employment was crucial to the family finances. Local social workers and health visitors in an effort to solve the problem worked together to recruit suitable voluntary help to care for such children during the mother's absence and to put mothers and helpers in touch with each other.

Imagination and combined effort applied to local problems can provide some of the solutions while others need to be referred through the system to the joint consultative committee so that joint funding and agreement on responsibilities may be reached.

RESPONSIBILITIES AND OBJECTIVES OF THE SCHOOL HEALTH SERVICE

1. *Responsibility to the child* To recognize and institute treatment for disorders likely to affect learning and social development throughout the school years.

2. *Responsibility to parents and teachers* To ensure that they are aware of the significance of such disorders to the child's learning and life generally.

3. *Responsibility to local education authority* To provide advice and services on all aspects of child health and particularly in relation to children in need of special education (Section 34 1944 Education Act).

There are indications from research surveys as to what this is likely to mean in an ordinary school. The Isle of Wight Survey[1] on the 9 to 12 age group findings were:

Intellectually retarded	2.6%.
Educationally backward	7.9%.
Psychiatric disorder	6.8%.
Physical disorder	2.7%.

Therefore, in a primary school of 250 children there are likely to be 6 to 7 children with a physical problem and about 17 children with a psychiatric problem. This, of course, will be influenced by the general social problems of the children and is likely to be much higher where there is poverty, poor housing and poor parental care. To achieve these objectives it is desirable that every school should have a nominated school doctor and nurse whose function is fully understood by the school and staff of the local education authority. There are many teachers who are very well informed. However, this is not always so and some know comparatively little about the role of the health team and the kind of help and service that can be offered. This probably stems firstly from the lack of emphasis on this aspect during teacher-training and secondly from their experience of the service in practice. Teachers seek help and co-operate largely as a result of contact with an effective school health service. Care and effort needs to be taken in planning the service to fully consider the teachers' needs and to cause the least possible disruption to the school curricula. Efforts also need to be made to take an active part in school life by participating in parent-teacher's meetings, social functions, coffee breaks and lunches, attending school sports and open days.

The necessity for good communications between the school health service and the school cannot be overstressed, particularly in large schools, and efforts should be made for the school doctor, school nurse and head teacher to talk together from time to time and seek solutions not only for individual children but for organizational problems such as poor attendance of parents at medicals or accommodation problems affecting the health service to the children.

Staffing

The service in individual maintained schools is provided by a school doctor and nurse, and the dentist and his team. They all need to work closely with the teachers, social workers, educational psychologists, education welfare officers and parents. Additional back-up from the health service comes, if required, from family practitioners, the appropriate hospital specialists, speech therapists, physiotherapists, dieticians and others.

At the present time the system of staffing and the training of personnel involved is under discussion and new proposals have been made by the 1976 Court Report.[2] These are designed around the concept of primary care teams which include family practitioners in group practice and attached nursing staff (including the school nurse) and social workers. However, even if these new proposals are accepted, it is unlikely that change can be immediately effected and a variety of patterns may be found for some years.

The school doctor The doctor will be a key figure in the school, overseeing the health of the children and providing the education staff with information, advice and guidance regarding the management of health. Under the new proposals he may in the future also prescribe treatment which as we have seen has up to now been the prerogative of the family practitioner. Consequently, the school doctor has had to refer all children needing prescriptions. Sometimes, particularly in boarding schools, the school doctor may also be the child's family practitioner, in which case he will of course prescribe treatment.

In the past school doctors have not been required to take additional training unless they were involved in making recommendations for special education, when an approved certificate was required. Latterly, a course of one year's duration has been recommended. The service tended to be staffed by either doctors employed full-time on pre-school and school health work, or general practitioners on a sessional basis. Consequently, the level of service varied considerably according to the doctor's interest and understanding of child development.

Under the new proposals and in order to combine the screening and treatment service, the school doctor will be either a GPP (a general practitioner with a special training in paediatrics and child development and whose work in group practice is mainly with children), or he may be CHP (a child health practitioner, also with special training but appointed by the area health authority and attached to a group practice, health centre or child health clinic). The school doctor in special schools will be a senior experienced doctor (consultant community paediatrician) who will also be a member of the district handicap team (see p. 24).

The school nurse The school nurse should be a good partner for the school doctor. Primarily, she should be someone who has a good rapport with children, as well as having had experience and training in the care of children during her nursing career. Her role includes consultation with parents and teachers, identifying and referring children in need of medical examination, following up the doctor's instructions and recommendations and encouraging and participating in health teaching; practical nursing procedures may need to be carried out in clinics or in school.

As we have seen, the 1945 Handicapped Pupils and School Health Regulations recommended that all school nurses should be qualified health visitors. However, there have never been enough health visitors and various staffing patterns have grown up throughout the country. To maintain continuity between pe-school and school years, the primary schools have usually been the province of the health visitor while SRNs have been appointed to service the other schools. Sometimes they have been appointed full-time for school duties and have worked independently of health visitors and sometimes they have been given combined duties with child health clinics and have been responsible to the health visitor. Occasionally SENs have been employed similarly. Training for SRNs employed as school nurses was non-existent or provided on an in-service basis and varied from one authority to another.

The new proposals[2] recommend that a CHV (a health visitor with special training and expertise in child health) should have overall responsibility for a number of schools but that the day to day work should be undertaken by a specially trained school nurse with suitable background experience with children, who would either be required to be responsible for two to three schools, depending on the size, or she may be full-time in a large comprehensive school. The training should include child development, psychiatry, disorders that affect education, such as hearing and vision, together with knowledge about the education and social work services. The suggestion is that the Council for the Education and Training of Health Visitors should set up this course which should eventually lead to a Higher Certificate in Educational Nursing.

Nurses employed by boards of governors in independent schools or indeed by some local education authorities in maintained schools need to pay particular attention to their job descriptions which may include a variety of duties ranging from laundry and mending work to counselling the children. Usually school matrons are responsible for the day to day 'home' care of the children, including first-aid, while sanitorium sisters undertake sick nursing and sensory screening.

Also, it should be remembered that such service is not normally included for incremental advance when re-entering the NHS. To avoid professional isolation the nurse should enquire what arrangements she may be permitted to make for in-service training and it is quite possible, and indeed desirable, that agreements might be reached with the local area health authority for her to attend appropriate training courses and form links with the school nurses in their employment. The area nurse (child health) of the authority should be approached to advise and make arrangements.

The school dental service This is part of the school health service and is concerned with prevention, education and treatment. Like all health practice, patterns of good dental care and regular attendance established during childhood and school days are likely to be continued in adult life. The service is run by the area dental officer who is directly responsible to the area health authority. His functions is to assess the kinds of dental care likely to be required in the area, taking into consideration the type of local population and allocating resources accordingly. The school dental programme will be part of his plan for the whole area dental service.

The day to day service in the school is increasingly becoming a team approach, the leader of which is a qualified dentist who has undertaken a five-year course and is registered with the General Dental Council. He may be assisted by dental auxiliaries who have undertaken a two-year training and are also registered with the General Dental Council. Their training permits them to carry out certain treatments relating to dental caries and peridontal disease as prescribed by the dentist. They may also undertake the preventive measures of scaling and polishing the teeth, topical application of fluoride, and dental health education. Alternatively, this may be carried out by dental hygienists who have a nine-month training relating to the preventive measures only.

Dentistry is free to school children and a parent may elect to send a child to the family dentist for treatment or use the school dental service. The dental clinics are usually sited in large secondary schools, health centres or child health clinics and appointments are made either centrally or at the local clinic. Schools for severly handicapped children may have facilities sited in the school to avoid the difficulties associated with transporting the child and to have expertise of staff familiar with the children directly to hand.

There should be good communication between the medical and dental staff.

Many referrals will be made by the doctor as a result of medical examination or by the nurse following a health check. It is particularly important that medical details of illnesses or handicaps are made known to the dentist and that he is told of drugs that the child may be taking in case local or general anaesthesia is needed.

The dental policies on fluoride, oral hygiene, diet and topical applications of preventive agents should be known to the nurse so that she may reinforce the teaching when opportunities arise.

Back-up Health Services

The advantage of an integrated child health service is that the varying facets of the service can be more easily planned to dovetail and complement each other. The school doctor or general practitioner will refer children to appropriate specialists and departments as he thinks fit. Many district general hospitals now have comprehensive assessment centres where a wide range of specialist expertise and supportive therapy are available, including social and child psychiatric services. The approach is essentially multi-disciplinary and the aim is to achieve a full assessment of all aspects of the child's life so that a programme of care can be planned which will provide social support and practical advice to the parents, together with suitable medical treatment and education for the child. The plan is continually reviewed and future employment possibilites are kept in mind. This present nucleus of expertise will form the basis of the district handicap team if the 1976 Report of the Child Health Service is accepted. (Nursing will be represented by a nursing officer with special knowledge of handicap who can assist the health visitor and school nurse in providing better service to the parents.) The school health team can expect and should ask for information and guidance from them on the handling of the handicapped child in school.

Adolescents often need assistance outside the school to help them in their new decisions of adulthood. For this purpose 'walk-in advice centres' providing family planning information together with guidance on general problems of personal relationships, sex, venereal disease and abortion may be made available. Local facilities will vary considerably and it is necessary to establish at an early date what expert advice is likely to be available and where support services may be found.

Associated Services

Needs may not always be medical but are likely to be equally the province of the education service, the social services, housing departments, the juvenile courts, police and probation officers, or the environmental health department (see Fig. 4).

Environmental health As outlined at the beginning of this chapter, the environmental health and community medical and nursing services were a combined health service administered by the local authority until 1974. With reorganization the service was split leaving the environmental health responsibilities with the local authority. The present department, usually headed by a chief environmental health officer, is responsible for the control of infectious diseases, food inspection at ports and in shops, factories and restaurants, measurements of air pollution, control of vermin, unfit housing and drainage, and health and safety at work. They usually carry out these functions as they relate to schools on behalf of the education authority and will be particularly involved with the school health team in connection with infectious diseases and the school environment. They are closely associated with the health authority in that medical advice is given to them by the proper officer who is usually the district community physician.

Fig. 4. Support services available to the child in school and the various types of associated back-up services. Notice the demarcation lines between the services which need to be bridged.

Parent - teacher associations

EDUCATION SERVICE

Special educational facilities

Transport   School meals

Youth and careers services

Educational psychologist

Advisory teachers

School counsellors

Education welfare officers

Teacher

Social worker

Senior and specialist social workers (blind, deaf, handicapped, psychiatric)

Fostering, adoption and care supervision

Short-and long-stay residential homes

Liaison with voluntary organizations

SOCIAL SERVICES

Housing

Social security payments

Probation service

Police (Juvenile bureaux)

Magistrates courts (Juvenile panel)

THE FAMILY

Friends

Extended family (grandparents, aunts, etc)

Parents

CHILD

Community health councils

Voluntary services

MPs

Embassies

Environmental health services

Doctor

GP (GPP)*

Consultants (community, paediatric or specialist)

Therapists

Hospital departments out-patients; accident and emergency

In-patients; short- and long-stay

Dental hospital

Dental auxiliary or hygienist

Dentist

Nurse

HV (CHV)*

NO (CHV)*

Hospital nursing staff

HEALTH SERVICE

* Represent staff proposed by the Court Committee on Child Health Services, 1976

Housing department The provision of council housing is also a responsibility of the local authority. The department is headed by a director of housing and deals with the allocation of homes according to need and availability of accommodation. The dilemma he faces is usually that the demand is far greater than the number of homes his department has at its disposal. People are usually required to enter their names on a waiting list and accommodation is allocated as it becomes available, which in many cases may mean a wait of several years. Desperate need may, however, be given priority and a certain number of lettings may be reserved for families who need accommodation for health reasons. A school may be involved in negotiating with the housing department where it can be seen that the child is suffering considerably as a direct result of unsuitable accommodation which the parents are in no position to alter. This may be particularly the case where physical handicap is involved.

The provision of accommodation for homeless families was until recently the province of the social services but as no accommodation was available for them large numbers of families ended up in 'bed-and-breakfast' hotels, often unsuitable for their needs and costing vast sums of money. Responsibility has now been placed on housing departments and they usually employ social or welfare workers within their departments to assess each individual case and negotiate with the various other agencies involved with the family. Children from such families have often short-stays in schools and are particularly likely to have a range of difficulties.

Social services Social services are provided by local authorities and their present structure and responsibilities date in the main from the 1970 Local Authority Social Services Act. They are responsible for a wide range of duties of which children and their families are a part. They have special responsibility towards the single mother and her child, fostering and adoption, and services for the handicapped (1970 Chronically Sick and Disabled Persons Act).

They are likely to be involved with children whose parents are failing to cope for one reason or another: possible situations include intellectually subnormal parents, mental or physical illness of one or both parents, financial mismanagement, separation, divorce, death, re-marriage, criminal behaviour, violence and a host of other social upheavals. Social workers aim to help families solve or adjust to their problems but inevitably there will be occasions when the child can no longer remain in the home, in which case arrangements for foster care or adoption may have to be considered. Liaison with other agencies such as health, education, police or the courts, is an important aspect for success in their work.

To support them in their efforts to make satisfactory arrangements for the care of children, the registration of child-minders, play-groups and day nurseries (1948 Nurseries and Childminders Act amended by Section 60 of the 1968 Health Services and Public Health Act) are also the province of the social services department as well as the provision of foster homes and residential community homes. These are not all run and staffed by social services. Some will be run by voluntary organizations but registered by the social services department and are often used by them.

Some social workers are also responsible for working with groups such as youth groups while others are responsible for community work which means encouraging communities of people to be self-supporting for their needs. Schools are sometimes used as centres for both group and community work.

The central council for education and training of social work is responsible for social work training in all branches of the profession, including residential care. Graduates are required to take a one-year course; otherwise a two-year training is necessary following an education which must be at least to the standard of five 'O' levels and preferably 'A' levels. However, because of the pressure of work and the shortage of trained staff, some may not have gained such qualifications.

Juvenile courts These are concerned with making legal judgements to protect the interests of the child. When a young child is being neglected, ill-treated, in moral danger or beyond the control of his parents, various arrangements may be made according to the circumstances to see that the child's situation is improved. The child may be taken away from the home and cared for in a community home or by foster parents. Alternatively, he may be left in the home but a suitably qualified professional worker, usually the social worker, will have a legal right to visit regularly and supervise the care.

Adolescents may come before the court for truancy and juvenile crime, the number of which at present is increasing rapidly. The court usually requires a full social report and frequently the educational psychologist and child psychiatrist is also required to give evidence. Sometimes the school doctor may be asked to submit evidence and very occasionally a health visitor or school nurse. When such a situation arises, her senior nursing officer should arrange for her to talk to a solicitor and preferably attend a court hearing before the proceedings so that she will be familiar with it.

Members of the public may not attend juvenile courts and the press are not allowed to publish either the names and addresses of those involved or the schools they attend. The kind of care which may be recommended for adolescents will vary. When a child is 14 years or over a probation officer may be required to supervise and as such may visit the school. Alternatively, arrangements may be made for care to be provided in one of the social services' special community homes which are gradually replacing the remand homes and approved schools which existed before the 1969 Children and Young Persons Act. A child found to be suffering from mental illness or psychiatric disorder may be committed to hospital for treatment.

Police The police are often the first to find children committing crimes, usually during periods of truancy from school. Such children may be released on bail to parents or placed in the care of the social services while the case is being investigated. The investigation and decision to prosecute is generally the decision of the juvenile bureau of the police department who will make enquiries about the family and the various agencies likely to know the child. From this the case may proceed to the juvenile court as described on p. 27.

Other services There are many other organizations who may be interested in the school children or who may be asked to assist for one reason or another. Some embassies support schools providing education on the lines of their own country for children of embassy staff or foreign nationals in this country. They may also provide advice when problems arise concerning children whose parents originate from their country but who have immigrated to Britain.

There are large numbers of voluntary organizations concerned, as a rule, with handicapped children. Local members of parliament and local councillors are usually interested in comments from the general public and may mediate on a distressed parent's behalf. Community health councils have a duty to represent the health needs of the public to the area health authorities and therefore should be interested to see that the best possible service is provided to children.

Nurses in schools need to make themselves aware of the functions of various organizations which may be involved with some unfortunate children, usually through no fault of the children themselves. This avoids mistakes and further injury to the child and is likely to improve considerably the quality of the nurse's own contribution to the growth and total development of each child.

REFERENCES

1. Rutter, M., Tizard, J. & Whitmore, K. (1970) *Education, Health and Behaviour.* Harlow, Essex: Longman.
2. Court Report (1976) *Fit for the Future—The Report of the Committee on Child Health Services.* London: HMSO, Cmnd 6684.

FURTHER READING

Annual Report of Chief Medical Officer (1971–2) *The Health of the School Child.* London: DES, HMSO.
Annual Report of Chief Medical Officer (1975) *The School Health Service: 1908–1974.* London: DES, HMSO.
Family Welfare Association—Guide to the Social Services. (Revised annually.) London: McDonald & Evans.
Fitzherbert, K. (1977) *Child Care Services and the Teacher.* London: Maurice Temple Smith.
Slack, G. L., & Burt, B. A. (1974) *An Introduction to Community Dentistry.* Bristol: John Wright.
Ruel Report (1974) *The Role of the School Nurse—Report of a Working Party.* London: Royal College of Nursing.

USEFUL ADDRESSES AND INFORMATION

The Council for the Education and Training of Health Visitors
Clifton House
Euston Road
London NW1.
Tel: 01 387 3456.

Responsible for the standards of health visitor training and in the future may be responsible for school nurse training if the recommendations of the Court Committee accepted by Parliament.

Can give up to date information on courses available and details of places, dates and cost.

The Association of Hampshire School Matrons and Welfare Assistants
Amery Hill Secondary School
Alton
Hants.
Tel: 0420 (Alton) 84545.
Mrs J. E. M. Allen (Chairman)

First association of its kind formed for purposes of mutual support and to provide opportunities for learning. Willing to advise other interested individuals or groups throughout the country.

Boarding Schools Association
90 Burbage Road
London SE24.
Tel: 01 274 9004.
Mrs J. G. Dewes (Secretary)

Run an annual 48-hour conference for school matrons and sanitorium sisters. Preference given to nurses from independent or maintained schools which are members of the Association.

Discussion Topics

1. You are going to an interview for a post as a school nurse. What information about the job would you feel it necessary to know before accepting the post, assuming it is offered to you?
2. At the local health centre you hear the health visitor and social worker

discussing the large number of children needing day care. However, there is a long waiting list for the day nursery and there are very few registered child-minders. You tell them that there are several vacancies in the nursery class of your school but they think that the hours are unsuitable to the parents' requirements. How might the joint consultative committee be used to solve this problem?

3. Discussion topic three at the end of Chapter 1 posed a problem about a child and his mother and you were asked to consider members of the education service who might be of assistance. Should any of the services or staff described in this chapter be involved?

4. Consider ways in which you might keep in regular contact with other school staff and add to their knowledge of the health service.

5. You are told that you may have to give evidence in court. What action would you take?

6. Consider the situation where there is a full-time school matron employed by the education authority and a visiting school nurse employed by the NHS. How might their duties complement each other and how could they work together to provide a first-class school nursing service?

3
Work Planning

The success and efficiency with which the nurse carries out her duties depends to a large extent on the use she makes of the accommodation available to her and the care with which she plans her work and sees that the clerical and recording duties are performed. The amount of help she gets varies from area to area and while everyone recognizes that it is not a good use of a nursing education to spend a large proportion of time on clerical duties, it is not always possible to obtain sufficient help. Whether or not duties are delegated, it is essential to be aware of good principles and see that they are followed.

Place of Work

Medical and nursing examinations are usually carried out in the school though a local health clinic or mobile unit parked in the school yard may be used where suitable accommodation is not available. Many older buildings have no purpose-built unit and an office, vacant class-room or assembly hall may need to be used for the purpose. Where such arrangements have to be made, the matter should be discussed with the head in good time, preferably before the term's curricula are decided, so that suitable rooms will be free as required. Failure to do this results in confusion and bad feeling. The nurse may find herself either with no accommodation in which to carry out her work or be allocated totally unsuitable rooms. I have known a nurse undertaking hearing screening to be offered one end of the assembly hall in which music practice was taking place. Under the 1973 NHS Reorganization Act, Section 3,[1] local education authorities and managers or governors of voluntary schools have a duty to make accommodation available for medical and dental inspections.

New school buildings should certainly have purpose-built medical rooms and where school populations are falling, consideration of the re-allocation of rooms should include the medical needs of the pupils. Where medical suites have been provided, they should be kept for that purpose and not be used as class-rooms or lunch-rooms. Ill children need to lie down or be quiet and first-aid may be required.

There is always a certain amount of administrative work associated with school health and time may be wasted if the medical room is found to be occupied. Parents and pupils are probably more likely to use the service if there is an established 'health territory' and the times at which the doctor and nurse are available are well known in the school. This information can be shown as a notice on the medical room door or the general school notice board, and printed in the school information handbook distributed to parents and pupils.

The medical suite incorporating accommodation for the doctor, nurse and dentist should be situated in a quiet part of the school with easy access to toilets. There should be comfortable accommodation for parents to wait and changing rooms where children may undress in privacy: this is particularly important in the secondary school. There should be adequate space for the doctor and nurse to function independently of each other but be within easy calling distance. Rooms should be large enough and sufficiently well-lit to enable vision screening to be carried out satisfactorily; a sound-proof area is necessary for hearing testing. A wash-basin in each room and locked filing and storage space should also be provided. There should be somewhere for an ill child to lie down and for first-aid to be administered. To facilitate communication, consideration might also be given to the proximity of the medical accommodation to the rooms provided for school counsellors, social workers, educational psychologists and the head teacher. Figure 5 illustrates a suggested plan for a primary school; it enables doctor and nurse to function independently, and first-aid or nursing for a handicapped child may be given without interfering with the medical. A sick child can rest in the changing/rest room and be observed by the nurse or secretary. A secondary school would require more space and would include dental accommodation.

The following equipment is necessary:

1. Weighing scales, height measure and standard growth charts (metric conversion tables if necessary) and transparent ruler for use in charting.
2. Vision screening equipment—as indicated by local policy—for distance, near and colour vision testing.
3. Tape measure and head circumference charts.
4. Picture books, toys and drawing paper and developmental testing materials as required by the doctor.
5. Stethoscope, auroscope and torch (as necessary—many doctors prefer to use their own).
6. Full range of area health authority school health stationery.
7. Reference material, i.e. telephone directories, street lists, local education authority school index, medical and nursing reference books, area health authority school procedures, family practitioner list.

Additional equipment for treatment may be required if Parliament accepts

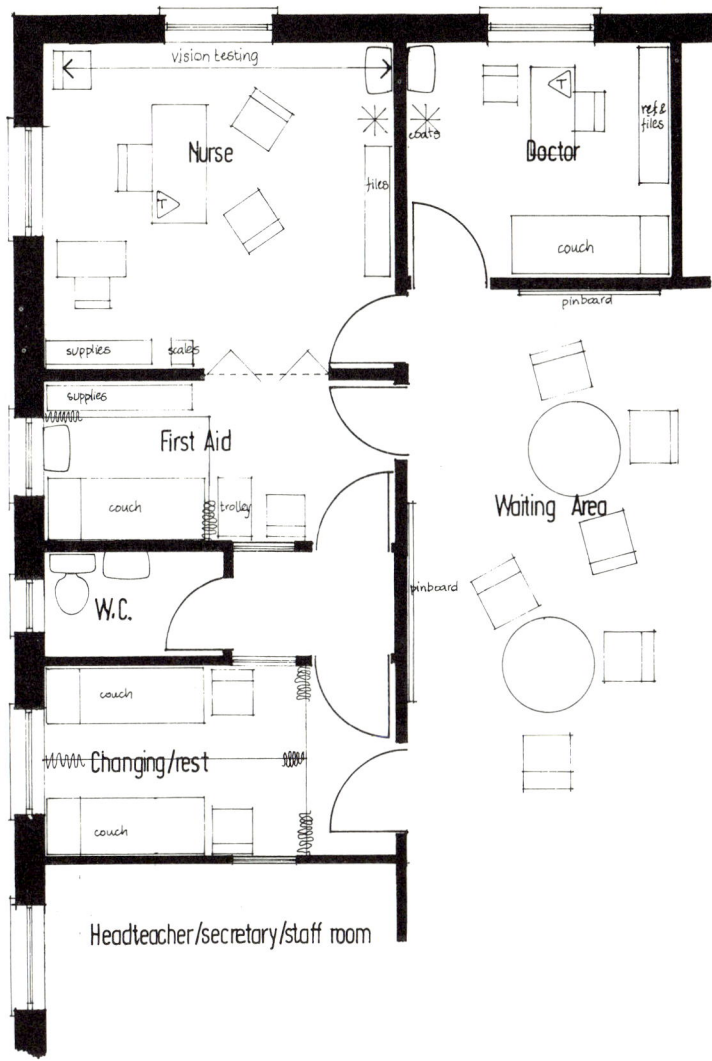

Fig. 5. Architect's impression of a medical suite for a primary school (c. 240 children).

the recommendations of the Court Report[2] thereby combining assessment and treatment in the school health service.

The organization of the medical room should reflect the needs of the children; young children are encouraged to relax and play in an informal setting while adolescents have the privacy and degree of professionalism that recognizes their young adult status.

Planning

Time spent on good planning is well worthwhile. It tends to clarify what exactly needs to be done and it establishes a routine which leads to greater efficiency and prevents mistakes and delay.

Job descriptions and check-lists provide a basis from which to make a list of everything that should be done throughout the year. From this the number of medical and nursing sessions needed in the school can be calculated by adding up the time required to complete each task. Broad national guidelines such as 6 hours nurse time per week (primary school with 240 children) and 15 hours nurse time per week (secondary school with 1000 children)[2] can only be a guide as the time needed will vary according to the state of health and development of the children and the ease with which their particular problems can be dealt with. Much more time is likely to be required in schools where a large proportion of the children come from deprived or disadvantaged homes.

Where the number of sessions required exceeds the number you can afford to spend in the school, the matter should be discussed with the nursing officer. Perhaps two sessions can be combined, for example, medical examination preparation and medical examination. Help may be available or, if this is not the case, priorities will need to be set for the order of importance of various screening and other tests. Such priorities should be fully discussed with the school medical officer and the difficulties made known through nurse management to senior nursing and medical staff at district or area level.

Having decided the number of sessions required for various activities, a target date should be set for their completion. Plan around this, taking into account the most suitable time of day, term or year; for example home visiting, filing and record work might be allocated to holiday periods, hygiene surveys to the beginning of term when children are most likely to be infested, and medical examinations to the middle of term when children are most settled.

Where several schools are involved, visits should be planned so time is not wasted either travelling from school to school or on long journeys between home visits. Two diaries should be kept, one to remain at base so that appointments may be made on your behalf and to provide information as to your whereabouts. Details of time, place and task should be entered in the diary so that in the event of your absence, alternative arrangements can be made. If documents or equipment have to be taken from a central place, make a note in good time so that this can be organized. The diary may also be used to enter time spent on each activity. This information may be used to help future planning or to provide evidence to senior staff for the need of extra help or time in school.

Communications

Good communications are extremely important if work is to be effective. No one person can take appropriate action on every problem and satisfactory arrangements need to be made for passing on information and discussing plans and difficulties with teachers, doctors, social workers, parents and other colleagues. Contact may be made in the following ways.

Personal contact This is by far the most effective method of communicating and it is generally advisable to make personal contact initially with everyone with whom there will be a need to work closely. First meetings can be very important as it may be difficult subsequently to change a bad impression. Teachers may not appreciate the role of the school nurse so it may be useful to outline those aims which relate closely to the colleague in question and also to outline areas where co-operation will be valuable. This enables each party to have a clearer idea of the other's role.

Arrangements may be made for regular meetings or the nurse may be invited to attend as appropriate. Intermittent difficulties can be discussed at ad hoc meetings of those concerned but when the problems of individual children and their families need discussion, a case conference may be called (see p. 52).

All meetings should be planned and prepared, whether they are on a one-to-one basis or for a larger group. The reason for meeting and the items for discussion should be made clear, either informally when an appointment is made or by the issue of an agenda which enables those concerned to assemble relevant information and to prepare questions which may be of mutual concern. If someone cannot attend a meeting, it should be cancelled unless the absentee can provide written information relevant to the agenda. A meeting should not be allowed to take place if the absence of one person renders it valueless. Meetings with parents are likely to be on an individual basis in the school or at the child's home (see p. 134). Preparation for this kind of meeting is equally important and a few brief notes in a diary or note-book can serve as a reminder that all the necessary points are covered.

Telephone This is a good and quick form of communication, second best to personal contact though there are certain disadvantages, in that conversations may be overheard and mistakes made with the identity of the person at the other end. Therefore, care must be taken that confidential information is not divulged to inappropriate people. A note recording the date and time and any decisions should be attached to the appropriate file or record.

Written communication This usually takes the form of:

1. Internal memoranda.
2. Letters.
3. Reports.

These are generally made to confirm verbal agreements, make contact, give information, outline a problem for discussion or as a statement of a situation or incident.

Internal memoranda These are used to communicate with people working within the same department of the area health authority. They are generally circulated to several people, each initialling and dating the paper and passing it to the next person listed. They are usually conveyed by an internal delivery system in prepared re-usable envelopes provided for the purpose.

Letters Letters are used to communicate with colleagues in other services. A correct format should be used, i.e. address and date on top of the page, reference numbers for reply should be quoted to speed delivery and a subject heading enables the purpose to be clearly understood. Wherever possible address the recipient by name in which case the letter should conclude 'Yours sincerely'. The body of the letter should be clear and as brief as possible, yet contain all the relevant information. Typed letters are easier for colleagues to read and refer to later. A nurse must be able to draft a letter and to have it typed if necessary. Sometimes it is more appropriate to send a handwritten letter which is friendlier and tends to be less intimidating than a type-written letter which to parents signifies officialdom.

Reports A report is a written summary of a situation or problem setting out the relevant information, findings and conclusions, and sometimes making recommendations for action. They may be asked for by senior nursing or medical staff to enable them to take decisions on all sorts of matters. A typical example is a child with suspected non-accidental injury when a report is an automatic requirement. The subject should be clearly stated at the beginning and where families are involved the names, date of birth and address of each member should be tabulated. The information in the body of the report should be brief, logical and to the point, with conclusions clearly stated at the end. Where recommendations are required they should be tabulated clearly and briefly and some indication given of the possible consequences of their implementation.

The organization of secretarial and typing assistance varies and there may be occasions when it is necessary to dictate to a secretary or to use a tape-recorder. This takes practice and preparation for success. Simple rules are as follows:

1. Indicate the type of letter (memorandum, letter, report).
2. Number of copies required.
3. Name of the sender and the recipient, any references.
4. Heading.

Make rough notes so that all points are included and they follow a planned sequence. Medical terms should be spelt and speech should be clear and not too fast. A tape-recorder has the advantage that it can be stopped, re-played and rubbed out frequently without wasting anyone's time. Practice and instruction are needed initially and the typist herself is often the person to provide help.

Sometimes an accompanying slip is sent with the tape indicating the length of each letter, calculated from the figures on the recorder (for example: 0–5, letter to Joe Bloggs; 5–15, report to senior nursing officer; 16, correction: change Anthony Miller to Anthony Hopkins Miller).

Record keeping Accurate and comprehensive records can provide a total picture of a situation and how it has developed, either on a personal level for individual children, or as a statistical index to the service as a whole. Well-designed records should be simple to read and follow, require the minimum amount of writing to complete and be easy to file and re-order. Systems for re-checking and follow-up should be built-in so that time is not spent transferring piecemeal information from a number of books and files. Records and information systems need to be uniform throughout the area so that relief or peripatetic staff know exactly where and how to find information and to leave accurate up-to-date information on concluding their work.

The design of pre-printed stationery, the area records and systems will be the responsibility of an administrator who should be able to offer help and advice and may welcome suggestions for improvement.

Medical records A child's school medical record should be a comprehensive account of his general development and medical history, including illness and treatment throughout his school life. The pre-school records are obtained from the health visitor before school entry and should be available at the new entrant medical examination. When a child transfers from one school to another the medical record is also transferred. Parents do not always know when they are moving or tell the school; therefore the onus for requesting records rests with the area health authority responsible for the receiving school. Families returning from abroad may have records from a previous address in Britain or from SAFFA, if they are children of men in the armed forces. Any failure in the system of recording or passing information must be notified to the nurse management at once. Medical examinations and decisions taken in the absence of the previous history may be incorrect and not necessarily in the interests of the child. Maria Colwell's death was a tragic illustration that it is frequently the child most at risk for whom there is no previous record available. A national standard school medical record no. M10 is available from Her Majesty's Stationery Office and is still used by many area health authorities, although it is somewhat out of date. Other forms are being used experimentally either as part of a manual or a computer system and a working party set up by the Department of Health and Social Security (DHSS) is developing a new national standard system for child health records. The system designed for computer is divided into three parts which include a basic child register linked with immunization, pre-school health 0 to 5 years, and school health 5 to 16 years which will be the last to be developed.

The school medical records may be kept in a number of places, in the school clinic, by the area specialist in child health, by the district community physician, or in the medical room in the school. The information is confidential and should be kept in secure locked storage with access only by the school doctor or nurse, though arrangements must be made for the head teacher to be informed of matters relevant to the pupil's performance and general welfare. Standard national records still in use:

Form 10M (boy) Form 10M (girl)	Main school medical record used for pupils in all main-tained, primary and secondary schools, including special schools.
Form 10aM (boy) Form 10aM (girl)	Main school medical record—continuation sheet.
Form 10bM (boy) Form 10bM (girl)	Subsidiary school medical record kept so that day to day matters such as absence due to illness, inspections or other medical events can be recorded in the absence of the 10M. This information should be transferred as soon as the 10M is received.
Form 11M (boy) Form 11M (girl)	School dental record—usually kept in dental clinic attended by the pupil.
Form 12M	Medical records envelope in which the other records are kept.

Filing A good filing system should enable information to be found quickly and easily. There are a variety of methods, the vertical one being generally used for school medical records. They can be placed in sequence either (1) alphabetically (by name)—by far the most common method (2) numerically (by date of birth, or NHS number) (3) geographically (by class-room—of little use in schools where children are constantly changing classes or where there is a high turn-over of children).

To save time, papers such as notes, messages, letters received or copies of replies may be collected together over a period of days and then sorted into filing order and added to each individual file. When records are borrowed or removed from the cabinet, they should be replaced by a tracer card bearing the name of the borrower and the date. Similar cards may be used to indicate records requested and not yet received.

The names of individual children needing re-checking at varying times may be recorded on follow-up cards filed in a separate index. This can be divided into calender months and days 1–31. The cards can then be filed under the appropriate date and moved or refiled as the check is made.

Records need to be reviewed yearly, usually at the end of the summer term or in the school holidays. Old, unused, or unrequested records are generally stored. As the school health service changes in organization, records may be returned to the family practitioner or in certain circumstances passed to the Employment Medical Advisory Service. Disposal of records is controlled by the 1958 Public Records Act and in general medical and nursing records may only be destroyed six years from the date of the last entry unless it seems likely that they may be relevant in court proceedings. Further information regarding legalities of records may be obtained from the Public Records Office.

Statistical records Numerical information is required to monitor the service. Assessments may be made to find out whether all commitments have been met and comparisons can be made from year to year and with the services provided by other authorities. From this information plans are drawn up for future years and money and staff are allocated according to the needs shown by these figures.

Various methods are used to collect this information. At present the nurse is usually required to complete certain forms after each session, these being collated centrally by means of codes and punch-cards. This can be time-consuming and as computer recording develops it is likely that the child's personal record will be designed in such a way that certain information can be duplicated or detached and fed directly into the computer.

The opportunities for computers are immense but they are machines and only operate at the level of efficiency of the humans who design the programmes and, just as important, those who complete the forms and provide the information. So if the answers are misleading or inaccurate we must ask whether the information was fed in complete and correct.

Nurses all too often regard the submission of figures as a boring chore and miss the personal use which can be made of them in planning their own work and in evaluating their own efficiency and methods. Good returns should be carefully completed, show an accurate picture of the work and be used for future planning at every level. They are even more useful when considered in conjunction with education statistics such as the school population, age-grouping, and predicted trends as to the rise or fall in population.

Personal use A monthly, quarterly or annual break-down of the figures for each school with comparison and comment may be available. This is unlikely in this country at present and it will fall to the nurse to keep account of figures she needs. For example, the average number of children who require medical re-examination, fail vision screening, audiometry, or are referred for special examinations, may be used for planning the number of medical examination sessions needed (as outlined on p. 34).

Similarly, individual figures may be matched against national or local figures and discrepancies questioned, for example, if 7% of new entrants are thought to have a vision defect nationally, why are there only 1% in your school? Is it because the screening is not properly carried out or have the children really got better vision?

Nurse management use Management structures should exist to improve the service and working efficiency of the staff. The individual nurse's returns will show how she has allocated and spent her time and how productive her activities have been. They should indicate whether help is needed and possibly further training of the staff. The problems reflected in individual schools can act as a guide when recruiting staff; for example a school with a large percentage of children with behaviour problems might benefit from the assistance of a nurse with a child psychiatry training.

Further use The area, region, DHSS and World Health Organization will each use these figures for purposes of future planning, administration and evaluation. Around these figures buildings, equipment, staffing and financial allocation are planned. Scarce resources are used where special needs are indicated. Figures from other sources such as the Home Office, Department of Employment and DHSS are also used in connection with health planning and organizations such as the Office of Health Economics predict trends and highlight areas of special concern.

Local authority education departments use school health figures in planning buildings and equipment for special schools and classes. The present DHSS statutory returns on school health are as follows:

Form 8M (iv)	Screening tests for vision and hearing.
Form 8M (iii)	Eye diseases (defective vision and squint); diseases and defects of ear, nose and throat; orthopaedic and postural defects; diseases of skin; speech therapy; other treatment (minor ailments, recuperative holidays, BCG vaccination).
Form 8M (i)	Periodic medical inspections; other inspections (special and re-inspection); infestation with vermin.
Form 28M	School dental clinics; inspections; visits; courses of treatment; orthodontics; dentures; anaesthetics; dental health education.
Form 20M	Number of school clinics, for example, audiology, minor ailments, etc; child guidance clinics.
Form 28aM	Dental auxiliaries; dental hygienists.

Evaluation This takes place in part through the interpretation of the statistics just discussed, and review of the method and effectiveness of the work should be a continuous process. Changes need to be considered, tried and tested, before being instituted. Nursing is becoming more research-oriented and new methods based on this may be introduced or adapted to school circumstances.

Nursing in schools or indeed any non-medical institution can isolate a nurse from the profession, making it more difficult to keep up-to-date with changes and new ideas. The nurse has a responsibility to herself and her work to see that she is aware of developments, both in the nursing and medical professions and in the education service. Sources of information are numerous, including magazines supplied by the local education authority and by the health authority to local child health clinics. Local libraries, both adult and children's, may be sources of information, and specialist libraries usually admit visitors or will make suitable arrangements for books to be borrowed. Librarians are usually only too delighted to be of assistance.

Educational radio and television frequently plan a series of programmes for professional staff dealing with children in a variety of situations, including the school and the home. Many adult education institutes also run suitable courses for which employers are often willing to pay attendance fees.

Nurse management has a responsibility to see that information reaches the staff and that suitable arrangements are made to improve the skills of nurses in special aspects of the job through in-service training. Outstanding needs may be brought to the attention of management particularly at staff appraisal sessions.

Nursing research in Britain in the context of school work is practically non-existent at present and, therefore, presents an exciting prospect for nurses interested in this aspect of the profession.

REFERENCES

1. *National Health Service Reorganization Act* (1973). London: HMSO.
2. Court Report (1976). *Fit for the Future—Report of the Committee on Child Health Services*. London: HMSO, Cmnd 6684.

FURTHER READING

Butterworth, N. (1974) *English for Business and Professional Examinations*, 2nd ed. New York: McGraw Hill.
Davies, J. B. M. (1975) *Preventive Medicine: Community Health and Social Services* 3rd ed. London: Baillière Tindall.
DHSS (1975) *School Health Services—Records and Statistical Returns*. London: DHSS, HSC(IS)5.
DHSS *Standard Child Health System, HN 76*. London: HMSO.
Secretan, L. (1972) *How to be an Effective Secretary*. London: Pan Books.
The Standard of School Premises Regulations (1972) Statutory Instruments No. 25051. London: HMSO.
Walley, B. H. (1968) *Manual of Office Administration*. London: Business Publications.
World Health Organization (1971) *Statistical Indicators for the Planning and Evaluation of Public Health Programmes*. WHO Technical Report Series 472. Geneva: WHO (available HMSO).

USEFUL ADDRESSES AND INFORMATION

The Keeper of Public Records
Public Records Office
Chancery Lane
London WC2.
Tel: 01 405 0741.

Educational Broadcasting Information (30–BC)
BBC
London W1A 1AA.
Tel: 01 580 4468.

Run courses for professionals and also parents. Often have accompanying literature. Will send advance information on request or it may already be available in the school or adult education institute attached to the school.

Open University
(London region)
9 Grosvenor Street
London W1.
Tel: 01 499 0115.

Offers many courses in educational and environmental health studies suitable for nurses in schools. Guides to applicants are available from:
The Admissions office
The Open University
P.O. Box 48
Milton Keynes
MK7 6AB.

Discussion Topics

1. You are finding it very difficult to obtain the previous medical records of new entrants. What action would you take?

2. You have very little clerical help and find the completion of statistical returns takes a lot of time and the information is often repetitive. What would you do?

3. You have several children in the school with handicaps about which you know very little and have had no previous nursing experience with these conditions. How would you ensure that you are giving adequate nursing cover?

4. The number of classes in the school has been increased and you arrive one morning to find the medical room has been taken over for an extra history class every Thursday morning. What do you do?

5. There is no medical room in the school in which you work and it is impossible for the nurse and the doctor to function independently on medical examination days although this would be a more efficient way to work. You also notice that the numbers of children in the school are decreasing. What action might you take locally in the school and what action would you expect senior nursing staff to take in assisting you?

6. You are unable to complete all the duties required of you. How might you assist senior nursing staff in presenting evidence as to the need for assistance?

4
Medical Examinations

School medicals do not begin in a vacuum: they are a continuation of the pre-school surveillance started during the antenatal period and continued throughout the pre-school years by the health visitor and the family practitioner or child health doctor. Some children who enter the nursery school or class may have their pre-school surveillance carried out in the school either by the health visitor or the school nurse using pre-school documentation.

As soon as the health visitor knows which school the child will be attending she should transfer the pre-school record of developmental examinations together with a summary of her visiting into the school medical file, or if the child is attending a school in another area health authority the records should be forwarded to the new authority. Children of highly mobile families or circus or gypsy groups may have moved into the area and be unknown to the health visitor. Such children can be identified when the school issues a list of new entrants to the school nurse (usually during the term before entry). The present home address will, of course, be known to the school, and the health visitor or school nurse will need to see the parents to establish any previous addresses so that the early records may be traced. Any younger siblings will, of course, be of interest to the health visitor.

The nurse, in consultation with the school staff, normally has to select which children will see the doctor at each school medical session. Children may need to be seen for the following reasons:

1. New entrant examination ($4\frac{1}{2}$ to 5 yrs or new pupil with no previous school medical history).
2. Selective medical (requested by doctor, nurse, teacher, social worker or parent).
3. Assessment for special education.
4. Special examinations for
   a. employment,

    b. school journeys,

    c. admission or return to boarding school,

    d. candidates for higher awards, nautical courses and outward-bound schemes,

    e. recuperative holidays,

    f. infectious diseases,

    g. research investigations.

5. Secondary school medical examination (13 years or puberty).

1. New Entrant Examination

This examination is extremely important in that it should provide the teacher with enough information about the child's general development, weaknesses and strengths to enable the curricula and individual school work plans to be designed with them in mind. Strengths may be built upon, and weaknesses helped and supported.

At present this examination usually takes place when the child has been in school for one or two terms and has had sufficient time to settle down. This gives the class teacher time to get to know the child and formulate her own impression of speech, language, general abilities and behaviour. The doctor will wish to have these observations, and documentation may be available for the class teacher to complete, though this should not preclude direct discussion about any child with whom there is special concern. Similarly, relevant social information will be known to the education welfare officer. Perusal of the records and discussion with the health visitor will indicate to the school nurse which children have problems and arrangements may be made for these children to be examined on dates when the health visitor will be able to discuss the background with the school doctor.

Screening examinations for vision and hearing (see Chapters 5 and 6) together with measurements of height and weight, head circumference, and sometimes a urine test, should be completed by the nurse before the medical examination (see Chapter 9). The parents' co-operation is vital and arrangements should be made for one or both parents to attend with the child. The examination usually takes 20 to 30 minutes to complete, depending on the amount of information available in advance and the co-operation of parents and the child. The doctor will want to discuss some aspects of the child's development with the parents. The success of this type of examination depends to a great extent on the child's co-operation and so it is important that he is relaxed and confident. This can be encouraged by providing an informal comfortable atmosphere in the medical room and encouraging the child to examine the play material and explore his surroundings while the doctor talks to the mother. Examination will include discussion of the points outlined in the following sections.

Background history
1. Social and family: previous information from health visitor and education welfare officer; current situation and any familial handicaps or illnesses.
2. Medical and obstetric: pre-school records; current status and any additional developments, i.e. admission to hospital or recurrent illness.
3. Developmental milestones: previous records; additional information from mother.

Physical development *General appearance and growth*—doctor's observation; nurse's measurement of height and weight plotted on standard centile chart (see p. 126); head and face, including eyes, ears, skin and hair; heart and lungs; skeletal growth and posture; abdomen and genitals; *gross motor control*—walking, hopping, jumping or kicking a ball; *fine motor control*—finger and thumb grasp, building towers or bridges with wood blocks, writing and drawing; *performance of daily activities*—dressing, washing, eating, using the lavatory.

Sensory development Hearing and vision tests completed by nurse before medical.

Neurological development Laterality of hands and eyes, i.e. the dominant hand and eye; auditory memory; language development, including comprehension, expression and articulation; involuntary movements of face and hands; attention-span.

Psychosocial development Personality; relationships with other members of the family and school children; self-concept from mother's and teacher's observations. A wide variety of tests may be used and the skilled doctor gradually builds up a picture of the child's ability. The parents should be given some explanation of all this and if necessary reassured about the child or given some constructive advice how to best encourage him. The class teacher will need to know the doctor's observations, particularly if there is concern about any aspect of development. To back up this information, documentation relevant to the teacher's needs should be available for completion by the school doctor. This should be up-dated each time the child is examined so that the teacher may easily check his progress.

2. Selective Medical

Until recently, routine medical examinations were made on children usually at five years, seven years, eleven years and before school-leaving, and indeed it was compulsory under the School Health Regulations before 1959 that every pupil had not less than three inspections during his school life. Most authorities are now adopting selective examinations so that more time may be spent with the children who require it. Since 1974 the school entrant medical examination has not been a statutory requirement although there are proposals that, in view of its importance, it should be. There is also a proposal that in circumstances where a head teacher feels extremely concerned for the child's health and welfare a medical examination may be carried out without the consent of the parent, for example if non-accidental injury is suspected.[1] Such measures would require an Act of Parliament before they could be adopted.

These types of examination vary in the method of selection. Children needing follow-up are identified by the doctor at the new entrant medical and are seen again for review. Additionally, the parent, teacher, education welfare officer or the nurse, as a result of the annual health check, may consider that a further medical is required and so these children will also be seen. Some authorities send questionnaires to parents at regular intervals and children are selected as a result. The disadvantage of this method is that many parents are unable to read, fail to return the questionnaire or complete it inaccurately. There will, of course, be areas where none of this applies and this method may be very successful. Before selective medicals the nurse will need to check that all action or reports required from the previous examination are up-to-date and available and that yearly screening has been completed.

3. Assessment for Special Education

Children who are mentally or physically handicapped require special arrangements for their education which should start by the age of five years. Some children with a handicap may be able to cope in an ordinary school and, following consultation between the doctor, psychologist, parents and the head teacher, they will enter school with the other children; their progress must be followed closely to see that the placement is successful and that they are not either falling behind or indeed needing more than a fair share of the teacher's attention. The new entrant examination and subsequent selective examinations will identify children who are less obviously handicapped but who nevertheless have difficulty in keeping up in ordinary school and who require special attention in one way or another. Decisions then have to be made as to what kind of special help a particular child needs and how and where this kind of assistance may best be given.

These are very important decisions which may affect a child's whole life and consequently they need careful consideration and consultation with a range of experts. (A more detailed account of this is outlined in Chapter 8.) This kind of examination usually takes quite a long time and should be undertaken by a senior doctor experienced in such assessments. A separate session may be required for the purpose or assessment may be carried out over a period of time at a special assessment centre.

4. Special Examinations

These may be required for a number of reasons, the most common of these include the following:

Employment Children over 13 years are allowed to work outside school hours and frequently undertake newspaper rounds and Saturday or holiday jobs. In general a child may take a job for not more than two hours per day between 7 a.m. and 7 p.m. on Sundays and school days, though not during school hours. They may work up to eight hours on Saturday. Local bye-laws may impose further obligations on employers such as a certificate signed by a doctor before the child is allowed to work. This is usually completed by the school doctor.

School journeys Nowadays travel abroad is frequently part of the curriculum and it is necessary to check that children can undertake the journey and that the staff in charge are equipped to cope with any emergencies. Teachers must give adequate notice of pending journeys so that relevant vaccinations are given in good time to be effective before the start of the trip and that any conditions needing treatment have been attended to. The teacher in charge of the trip needs to know of any children with medical conditions such as asthma, epilepsy or enuresis which might be aggravated by the journey or who need special medication, supplies or arrangements to be made. They also need to take suitable first-aid equipment and be warned of any extra precautions required, for example attention to hygiene in countries where cholera, typhoid or paratyphoid are still a problem. Details of travelling requirements are set out in two DHSS booklets[2].

The school nurse usually re-checks the children for any sign of infectious disease 24 to 48 hours before the journey. Any sickly child should be excluded unless the teacher and parents understand and are willing to accept the consequences of infectious disease in a party of children on holiday.

Local policies vary as to how special medicals for employment and holidays are conducted. If a child has had a recent medical examination it is unlikely that it will be thought necessary to recall the child unless some new problem has arisen. Consequently, the doctor may sign certificates following perusal of the medical record. When medicals are required during school holidays, arrangements may have to be made in local child health clinics and consideration given to how records can be made available if they are normally kept in the school.

Admission or return to boarding school Some boarding schools require a doctor's certificate to say that the child is free from infection before they will allow the child to return. This avoids the inconvenience of having to immediately exclude the child or risk an epidemic in the school. Whether this is a necessary precaution to take in every case is questionable and it is only necessary where parents are insufficiently concerned for the child or incapable of recognizing such conditions.

This certificate is usually issued by the family practitioner though where parents can ill afford his fee this can be arranged at the local child health clinic.

Candidates for higher awards, nautical courses and outward bound schemes
These types of activity involve considerable mental and physical endurance,
gradually built up over a period of time by fitness training. Medical examination and advice is needed to see that children are physically able to undertake
these activities and that the training is not adversely affecting them.

Recuperative holidays Children who are not very strong might benefit from rest,
fresh air and exercise at a holiday home run by the education authority or a
voluntary organization, and admission may be arranged by the doctor.
Similarly, arrangements for free milk over the age of seven years or special
transport facilities require a doctor's certificate.

Infectious diseases When a child has been excluded from school or has been
absent as a result of certain infectious disease, for example, meningitis, it is
usual to re-examine the child soon after return for any adverse effects which
might have resulted.

Research investigations These may be carried out in school either by medical or
education staff, or both. The nurse may be asked to assist in data collection in
which case she should make sure that the senior nursing staff have been
consulted and that the proposed project has been passed by the appropriate
ethical committees as well as receiving parental permission. A nurse may wish
to initiate research into some aspect of school nursing work in which case
advice needs to be obtained through senior nursing staff, the area nurse (child
health) and the regional research liaison officer.

5. Secondary School Medical Examination

To find oneself in the wrong job, unsuitable to one's personality or capabilities,
is an unhappy and stressful experience for the young adult. Fatal accidents may
be caused if young people with certain defects are employed on duties affected
by a disability which in other circumstances might be quite innocuous, a
colour-blind person, for example, matching electricity wires; an asthmatic
working in dusty conditions on an automatic assembly line. Additionally,
employer's time is wasted if staff are taken on who do not progress
satisfactorily.

Teachers and careers officers start planning for a child's future around the
age of 13 years and therefore a medical examination needs to take place at this
time to assist them. Special documentation is available: Form Y9 for normal
children and Form Y10 for handicapped children. These are completed and
passed to the careers officer to keep on file for reference. At present school
health records are not passed on to occupational health services though often it
would be extremely helpful to have such an account. This may develop in the
future.

ORGANIZATION OF MEDICAL EXAMINATIONS

Once it has been decided which children require medical examination, it is necessary to plan which sessions they should attend. This will depend on how the doctor and nurse like to work and what is most convenient for the school and the parents. It may be more appropriate to see children for new entry examinations at sessions separate from selective and special medicals, or it may be more convenient to combine the two. Whatever plan is adopted it should be as efficient as possible and cause the least possible disruption to the child's education. Arrangements need to be made for parents to attend and for them to give written consent to the examination.

The room should be arranged to suit the ages of the children. Young children need an informal atmosphere with suitable play material to encourage them to relax, while adolescents require the dignity of proper adult facilities with privacy to undress and talk to the doctor alone. Nursing time is now an expensive commodity and the length of time allocated to each child for medical examination is longer. A child and his parents may expect to receive 20 to 30 minutes of the doctor's attention for a full developmental examination; this must inevitably increase the number of medical sessions in the school and also raises the question of the nurse's role during examinations.

Many doctors and nursing administrators see the nurse's function as helping to administer some of the tests for gross and fine motor control. While this broadens the nurse's role considerably, the prime consideration must be that existing commitments, such as annual sensory screening, be fulfilled before undertaking work at present carried out by the doctor. Secondly, part of the value of the tests carried out by the doctor is in the observation of how they are performed. Therefore, if the nurse is to do this, she requires extensive training in child development.

While it is obviously of the utmost importance that there is full communication between the doctor and the nurse and that the nurse is fully aware of the doctor's findings and the future plans for each child, it is undesirable that nursing skills are misused and time wasted. Provided that space allows, it would seem perfectly feasible to combine sensory screening and medical examination, for example.

Teachers object to continual disruption of classes as children are withdrawn on various occasions for screening procedures and medical examination, and this may also have the effect of making feed-back to the teacher disorganized and unco-ordinated. A more systematic approach would be less disruptive to the child's education, make more use of time available and be obviously more efficient and acceptable to parents encouraging them to attend future medicals and to consult the medical team on matters they are concerned about.

The following is a suggested sequence suitable for a primary school, combining preparation and medical examination, including immunization if the doctor is agreeable:

1. School secretary supplies new class-list at the beginning of each term.
2. Medical records requested from child health clinic.
3. *Three weeks* before the medical examination, nurse and head teacher discuss which children to request for examination, and school secretary enquires personally or by telephone whether this date will be convenient for one or both parents to attend. Nurse or education welfare officer, as appropriate, visits parents unlikely to show interest and explains the importance of the medical.
4. *Two weeks* before, consent forms and staggered appointments for medicals sent out by school secretary. A medical record is prepared for any child with no previous notes.
5. *One week* before, nurse checks medical records, immunization state, audiometry record, etc., completes and records preparations if unable to combine sensory screening and medical; sees that teacher' and social worker's reports are complete and ready and that consent form has been signed and returned.
6. *On the day*

   1.45 p.m. First child sees nurse: height and weight recorded; vision tested (distance, near and colour). Gets mother to sign any immunization consent needed.

   2.00 p.m. Nurse has brief discussion with doctor. Introduces mother and child to doctor. (Doctor completes the medical record himself as he examines the child.) Nurse returns to see second child as above.

   2.30 p.m. Nurse has brief discussion with doctor and brings in second child. Takes first child and parent out; answering further queries the parent(s) may have. Tests third child.

   3.00 p.m. Discussion with doctor and brings in third child and parent. Takes second child out and tests fourth child.

   3.30 p.m. Discussion with doctor and brings in fourth child. Takes third child out. Tests fifth child.

   4.00 p.m. Takes in fifth child. Accompanies fourth child and parent out.

   4.30 p.m. Brings out fifth child and parent. Discussion with doctor on findings and follow-up required. Checks and fills in the statistical returns. Checks records for next week's medical during any spare moments.

Such a sequence would ensure that medical preparation and examination would be completed in one session instead of two, leaving more time available for nurses to carry out yearly routine screening on other children. Selective and other medicals may take between 5 to 10 minutes and therefore more children can be seen.

Follow-up

During the examination the doctor will have discussed the child with the parents or guardian and decided whether there is any defect requiring treatment or referral for further opinion. The need for staff concerned with the child to be aware of the doctor's observations has already been stressed. Therefore, at the end of the session, there should be discussion between the doctor, nurse, teacher and education welfare officer or social worker, if possible, so that each may be aware of the doctor's findings and any action which may need to be taken. The doctor will complete or up-date the teacher's information sheet and the medical records. Letters may have to be written to hospital consultants and to the general practitioner for information. For certain common referrals, such as vision defects, pre-printed stationery may be available to save time.

Should a child need referral and neither parent has attended the medical, it is then necessary to contact them when one or other collects the child from the school, or to write to them. Only when written parental consent has been returned to the school can the appropriate referral be made. Alternatively, the parents may wish to arrange their own treatment via the family practitioner. Where parents fail to reply, a follow-up visit should be made by the school nurse or education welfare officer to establish the difficulty and persuade the parents of the necessity to have the child examined.

Continual failure to attend appointments must be followed up at home by the education welfare officer or it may be more appropriate for the nurse to visit to explain the procedure, treatment and implications for the child. The child himself can often influence the parents to take action provided the doctor and nurse have explained what they are trying to do and the advantages of the treatment. The biology and health education teacher may also help, if appropriate, by including simple details of the objectives of treatment in their teaching. Sometimes the doctor may decide to follow up the child at a school clinic.

School Clinics

These originate from the early days of the school health service when there was a need to provide free treatment for school children. At one time orthopaedic, ear, nose and throat complaints, and a host of other problems, were dealt with, even to the extent of surgical operation, by doctors and nurses in these clinics. With the advent of the NHS, children were more likely to be referred to the family practitioner or a hospital clinic and in some areas there are very few of these school sessions now. This type of clinic does, however, have the advantage of providing a withdrawal area, often outside the school in the child health clinic or health centre, where school doctors can examine children with particular problems and talk to parents at a more leisurely pace. Where possible they should be held outside school hours so as to interfere as little as possible with the child's education. School doctors may ask specialist consultants to conduct the clinic or assist in advising according to the kind of complaint being investigated. In some instances the school clinic may be regarded as a substitute or outpost of the district general hospital outpatients. This is a good idea where practical as it provides a more relaxed and informal atmosphere away from the hustle and bustle of the hospital, as well as being less 'illness' oriented.

The range of clinics will vary enormously throughout the country, according to local need. Asthma, enuresis, allergies, obesity, vision refraction, ortho-paedic and foot complaints, skin diseases, ear, nose and throat investigations and special problems relating to particular ethnic groups may all be dealt with in some depth at these special school clinics.

Nurses may or may not need to be present at the clinic and where children from a number of schools are attending a clinic, only one nurse is likely to be involved. Consequently, information relating to children from other schools must be relayed to them.

The whole question of communication (see p. 35) is a difficult one and often children are referred to consultants or therapists and no constructive information is returned to the school. This is a pity as it means that in spite of referral the school staff are continuing to work without expert advice. The absence of follow-up from such referrals should be brought to the school doctor's attention so that the matter may be pursued.

Case Conferences

Some unfortunate children have multiple problems both at home and in school, and there may be a number of social and medical personnel involved with the child and the family. When this happens it is generally a good idea to call a case conference to discuss the entire situation and to formulate an agreed plan of action. There is usually a set local policy on the method of calling a case conference which avoids muddle and duplication. Normally, social services are responsible for arranging a conference, providing the clerical back-up and ensuring regular review. Any professional person, i.e. teacher, doctor, nurse, social worker, worried about a child or family may request them to call a conference. All interested parties should be invited to attend. This may include the social security officer, housing department, probation officer, a voluntary organization as well as members of the health, education and social services. Any member unable to attend the conference should send a written report to the chairman or leader beforehand. In order that all those working with the child and family are fully informed, they should all receive written con-firmation of the agreed plan of action following the case conference.

REFERENCES

1. Court Report (1976) *Fit for the Future—Report of Committee on Child Health Services.* London: HMSO, Cmnd 6684.
2. *Health Protection Notice to Travellers* (1975); *Communicable Diseases Contracted Outside Great Britain* (1972). London: HMSO.

FURTHER READING

James, F. E. (1970) *Educational Medicine*. London: Heinemann Medical.
Rutter, M., Tizard, J. & Whitmore, K. (1970) *Education, Health and Behaviour*. Harlow, Essex: Longmans.

CHILDREN'S BOOKS

Rockwell, H. (1974) *My Doctor* London: Hamish Hamilton. Picture book illustrating some of the basic equipment a doctor uses. Suitable for nursery classes in preparation for medical examination.
Wolde, G. (1972) *Thomas Goes to the Doctor*. Leicester: Brockhampton Press. Picture book describing medical examination. Suitable for nursery classes.

Discussion Topics

1. You are employed as a school sister in an independent school. Would there be any advantages in having a pre-school history and how might you set about making arrangements to obtain these?

2. Consider ways in which children might be selected for medical examination with a view to adopting the most effective system.

3. A particularly shy and withdrawn child is due for medical examination next week. Consider how you might prepare the child.

4. The school doctor likes you to be present in the room with him during the school medical examination. He asks you to play with the child and administer the drawing and block building tests although he repeats these again himself. In order to do this you have to complete your preparation screening at a separate session and you do not have sufficient time to complete annual checks on all the children. Discuss.

5. The school doctor makes a number of referrals to specialist consultants at the district general hospital and to the school clinic for allergies and enuresis. However, no information which is needed by you and the teaching staff is forthcoming. Consider possible reasons for this and how you might set about altering the situation.

6. Discussion topic 3 at the end of Chapter 1 posed a problem about a child and his mother. You were asked to consider members of the education service who might be of assistance and at the end of Chapter 2 you were asked to consider other staff and services who might be involved. Reconsider the situation and suggest how all these people might be brought together.

5
Vision Screening

Defects of vision are very common among school children and regular checks need to be made to ensure that no problem passes unnoticed. One sight test indicating normal vision is not sufficient as the difference in the rate of growth of the eye and the rest of the body is such that a test may produce a normal result on one occasion but not necessarily the same result a year later. The child is not likely to be aware of being unable to see properly and the difficulty usually comes to light because of the observations of the child's reactions or through a routine vision check. Neglected vision defect can result in general backwardness, dislike of school and perhaps ultimately truancy and bad behaviour.

The eyes are also important in establishing relationships and communication between people. We all know how disconcerting a squint can be as you can never be quite sure whether the person is looking at you or what his or her reaction is. A child who cannot see facial expressions, or smiles and tears, is unlikely to respond and may consequently be mistrusted or regarded as unfriendly. Trevor Roper in his beautiful book *The World Through Blunted Sight*[1] illustrates the effect of various visual defects on personality and fortunes of many famous families and people.

Physiology of the Eye

The eye (approximately 2.5 cm diameter) (Fig. 6) is a sphere, the white tough fibrous cover of which is known as the *sclera*. The transparent area at the front of the eye is the *cornea*, behind which is the coloured *iris*. This is made up of small radial and circular muscles which contract enabling the pupil or dark hole in the centre of the iris to increase in size thereby admitting the correct amount of light. The darker it is the larger the pupil is to admit as much light as possible and vice versa.

Behind the iris is the *lens* which changes shape to accommodate the light and focus it on the retina or lining of the eye. The retina is made up of tiny fibres, the ends of which are known as rods or cones. These control the degree to which the eyes are sensitive to light. Absence or deficiency of pigment or vitamin A will affect these rods and cones and consequently the sensitivity to light. The impulses which start in the rods and cones move through the many nerve fibres of the retina and join up to form the optic nerve which carries these impulses to the brain. The point at which the optic nerve enters the eye is known as the *blind spot* and is unnoticeable when both eyes are functioning normally. One part of the retina known as the fovea or yellow spot consists only of cones which transmit colour images to the brain.

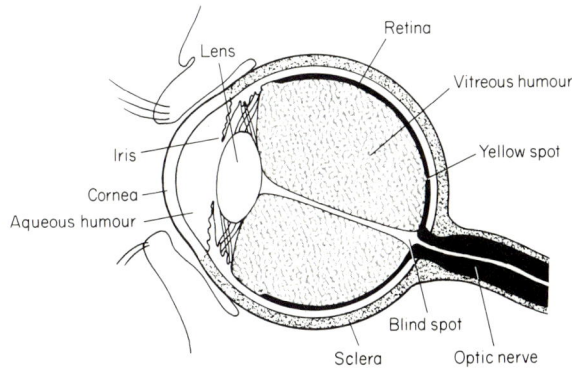

Fig. 6. Cross-section of the eye-ball.

The cavity between the lens and the cornea is known as the anterior chamber and is filled with a clear fluid called the aqueous humour. Raised pressure here results in glaucoma. The cavity of the rest of the eye behind the lens is filled with a jelly called the vitreous humour.

The common problems that the school nurse will encounter are usually those which arise when defects in the structure, such as poor shape, resilience of muscles, accommodation of the lens, and ability to distinguish colour normally are present.

Common Eye Problems

Refractive variations Rays of light are reflected from objects and are said to be refracted or change their angle as they enter the eye by the cornea and the lens. As people vary in shape and size, so do eyes and every eye will refract light and form images slightly differently. It is probably only when a degree of abnormality is great enough to hamper or curtail vision that treatment is required.

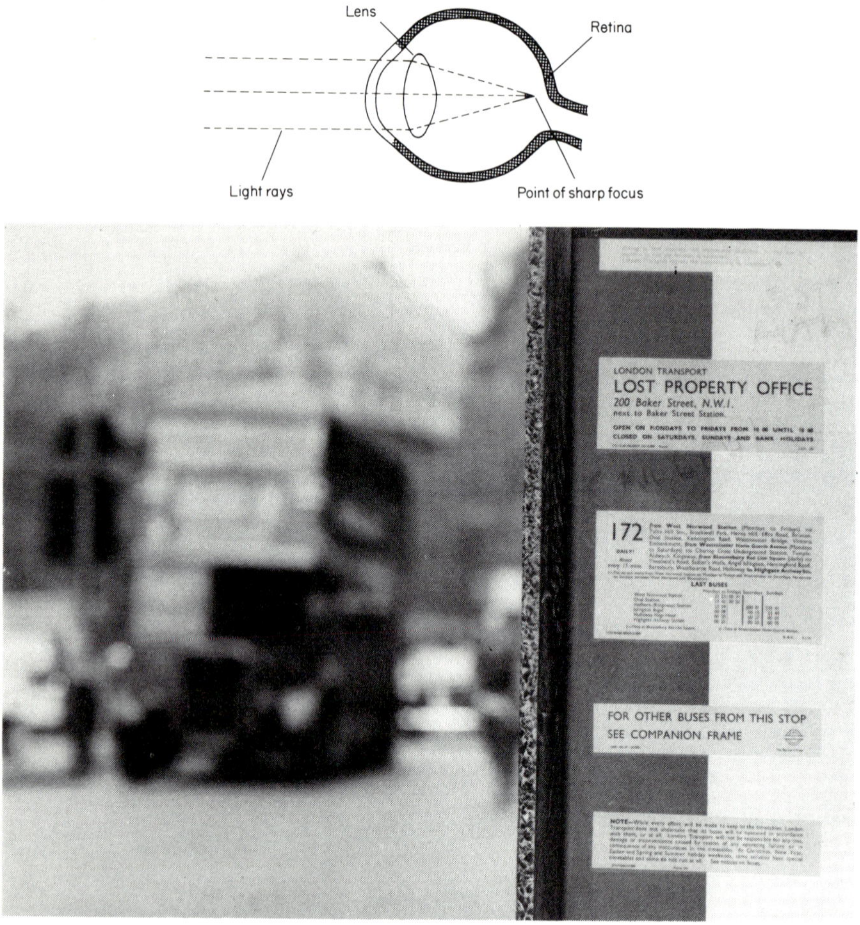

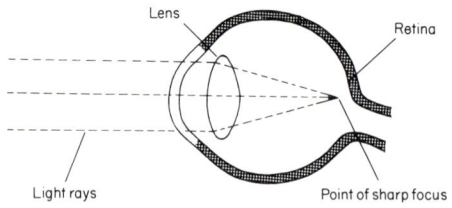

Lens
Retina
Light rays
Point of sharp focus

Fig. 7. Top: *Representation of myopia. In a myopic (or short-sighted) eye, light rays focus in front of the retina.* Bottom: *The reality of myopia. Short-sighted people can often see clearly at close range but do not have sharp vision in the distance. (Figs 7 and 8 by courtesy of the Optical Information Council)*

Myopia (short-sight) This is usually due to the eye-ball being slightly too long (Fig. 7). Children with myopia often have very large and beautiful eyes and the defect is most likely to become apparent about seven years of age or during a growth spurt such as puberty. Therefore, it is important to carry out a distance vision test at such a time. Handicapped children, particularly children with Down's syndrome, are frequently myopic and need regular vision screening and encouragement to wear their spectacles.

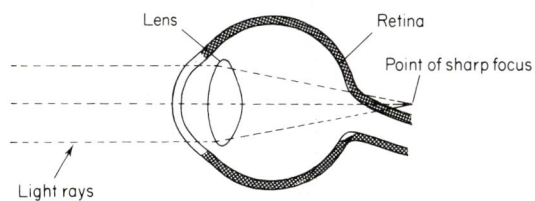

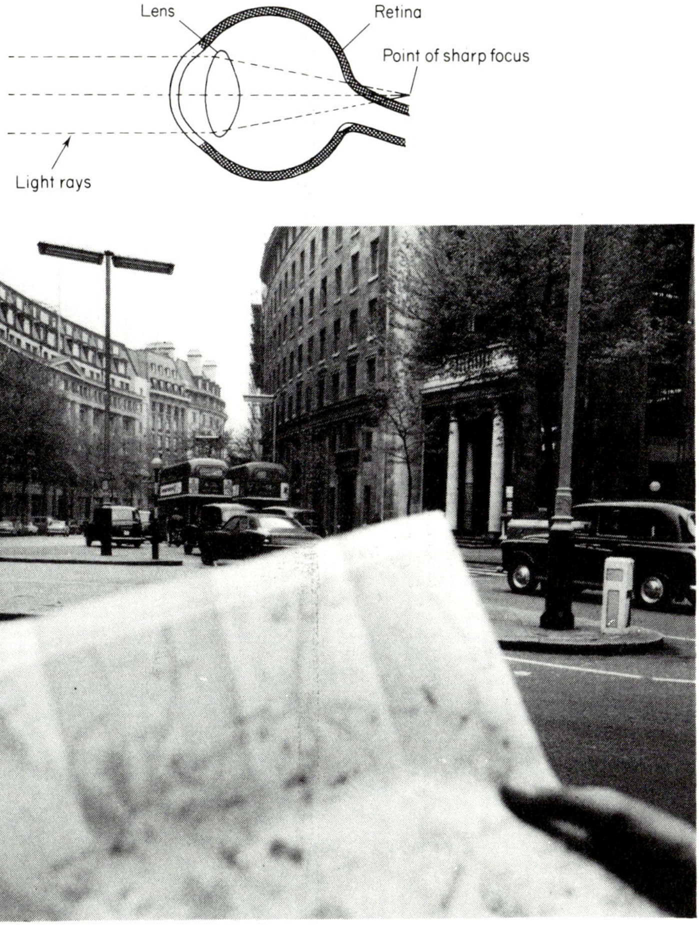

Lens   Retina

Point of sharp focus

Light rays

Fig. 8. Top: *Representation of hypermetropia. In a hyperopic (long-sighted) eye, light rays would, if they could, come to a point behind the retina.* Bottom: *The reality of hyper-metropia: clear vision at a distance and blurred details of the map held at close range.*

Hypermetropia (long-sight) This is when the eye-ball is slightly shorter and the eyes are usually smaller (Fig. 8). About half the population are long-sighted and it is normal in the young child. This is because the eye ball reaches full adult size relatively early in life; consequently, as the child grows the sight gradually improves. However, a child with a moderate defect will usually accommodate the vision sufficiently well to read though this may cause some nervous tension. Diagnosis is made by a near vision test which should be administered to every new school entrant.

Astigmatism This is a variation of the normal eye in which the curvature of the cornea or lens, or both, varies so that the images are distorted, usually making them appear vertically elongated. Astigmatism may occur alone or be combined with either myopia or hypermetropia.

Visual field defects Perfect vision includes being able to see all movements and objects within an area 190° horizontally, 70° upwards and 75° downwards, apart from the normal 'blind spot'. Vision may be restricted by other blind spots of varying size, shape and situation within these limits. It is more likely to be noticed because a child continually turns his head to the left or right in order to see better rather than to be noticed during routine distance and near vision screening.

Strabismus (squint, lazy-eye or cross-eye) This is a deviation of the direction of the gaze: a tendency for the eye to turn towards the nose is known as convergent squint; conversely, the eye turning outwards is known as divergent squint. This defect causes the child to have double-vision initially and to prevent this, the child eventually and subconsciously stops using the defective eye, resulting in a deterioration of the vision of that eye.

To ensure satisfactory treatment, diagnosis should be made before the age of five years, preferably before the age of two years. The degree of vision in each eye is tested and treatment in the form of exercises to train the eyes to work together is supervised by the orthoptist. Sometimes, treatment will also be accompanied by the good eye being occluded to exercise the lazy eye. This means that the child's vision may be severely impaired and the child will find the treatment unpleasant and resist it. Another difficulty is that as the treatment progresses and the eyes improve, the double-vision may return, distressing the child even further. Squint is a difficult condition to treat and it is best to discuss the matter with the orthoptist so that the school is fully conversant with the aims of the treatment. Surgery is sometimes indicated at an early stage but may be largely a cosmetic exercise to improve the look of the eyes and the vision in the weak eye may be lost.

Nystagmus This is a condition in which the eyes move about continually in an involuntary jerky fashion. It is usually present in both eyes and generally presents at birth or relatively soon afterwards.

There are two distinct types one of which may be herditary and, although there is no satisfactory treatment to stop the movements, the actual vision may be only slightly impaired. The second type may be associated with lack of pigment as in albinos, or congenital cataract or other conditions where the vision is severely impaired, for example it used to be common in miners working underground in insufficient lighting. Tinted contact lenses or glasses reducing sensitivity to light may improve the situation in selected cases such as albinism.

FREQUENCY OF TESTING

Ideally, children should be tested annually and every effort should be made to achieve this. However, this may not always be possible, in which case it is important to select children most likely to develop defects. They are as follows:

1. The child who is experiencing a period of rapid growth, or at puberty, usually between 7 and 14 years.
2. A child who already has a defect or handicap, for example rubella syndrome, cynotic heart disease, brain damage, Down's syndrome.
3. Family history of eye defect in parents or siblings.

It is also helpful to discuss the children with the class-teacher.

Any of the following observations might be an indication of short-sight and the child should have a *distance vision test:* bending closely over his books and desk work; unable to copy, reproduce or read anything correctly which is displayed at a distance, and may screw up his eyes in an effort to see it; dislikes or is bad at games such as hockey, football and tennis and seems clumsy, constantly tripping and falling over verges or small objects.

The following observations might indicate long-sight and a *near vision test* should be given: dislikes book work, irritable and complaining of headaches; inattentive in classes where close work or precision needed, as in some needle-work or crafts, while apparently enjoying games, films and projects where good long distance vision is required.

A *colour-vision test* would be indicated if a child constantly confused colours in art classes or was poor at a subject where colour graphs or illustrations were constantly used, as perhaps in mathematics, geography or history.

The following should be referred to the doctor:

1. Children constantly turning the head to the right or the left when looking at an object straight ahead or covering one or other eye.
2. All children with constant headaches, nausea or dizziness.
3. Any child producing mirror writing or spelling mistakes with the letters jumbled in the wrong order and spelt differently each time—this may not be a vision defect but dyslexia (as described on p. 91). Complete vision screening also needs to be carried out.

The brighter the child the more able he will be in compensating and functioning despite a defect. This needs to be remembered in all observations and tests.

Preparation

Vision screening may be carried out at a special session or combined with medical preparation or the nurse's yearly survey. Arrangements should be discussed with the head teacher. A suitable room should be made available if there is no satisfactory medical suite. Floor space of 6 m (20 feet) is required for distance vision test, or, alternatively, a mirror or reduced test cards may be used at a distance of 3 m (10 feet). There should be good lighting, plain decoration and no distractions or interruptions. Where conditions are unsatisfactory, the senior nursing and medical staff should be informed. The policy as to which tests to use and the frequency is decided by the area specialist in community medicine (child health). Nurses are unlikely to be required to test retarded children as this involves using materials suitable to the developmental age of the child. However, local policies may vary and special training to do this may be given.

Stycar (young children), Sheridan–Gardiner (5+ years) or Snellen (older children) tests are administered depending on the age of the child. Some authorities use a Keystone vision tester or Master vision screener which are designed to eliminate some of the adverse lighting and room conditions in schools. Whichever tests are in use the nurse should ensure that the instruction manual is carefully followed and any aspect which is unclear should be discussed with the doctor. Each time a test is recorded the name of the test should be entered as well as the reading.

Equipment suggested below should be gathered together beforehand:

1. Testing materials for distance and near vision, i.e. wall chart or seven and nine letter cards or books; alternatively, the Keystone apparatus.
2. Ishihara colour-vision set (should be kept in a box and not exposed to light other than when in use; one paint brush to use for tracing (fingers mark the book).
3. Children's school health records.
4. Notebook to enter any failures and the date of follow-up and any absent children.
5. Piece of unstretchable string, 6 m with a knot at 3 m (to measure the distance accurately).
6. An eye-patch, hair band or wooden spoon.
7. Piece of chalk (to mark floor distance).

Check with the teacher that each child recognizes and can say the letters of the alphabet and, if not, provide plastic letters or a key card for the child to indicate the letters seen: measure and mark correct floor distance; fix the eye chart at the child's eye level; talk to the child and examine the eyes, noticing the general appearance and any signs of blepharitis or conjunctivitis. Explain the procedure and if glasses are worn examine them for scratches and cleanliness, taking notice as to whether the fitting is comfortable. Children grow quickly and the frames may soon become too small. Test the child firstly without the glasses and then again wearing them.

Distance vision Occlude the left eye first making sure that there is no pressure on the eye ball as this may cause difficulty in focusing when the pressure is

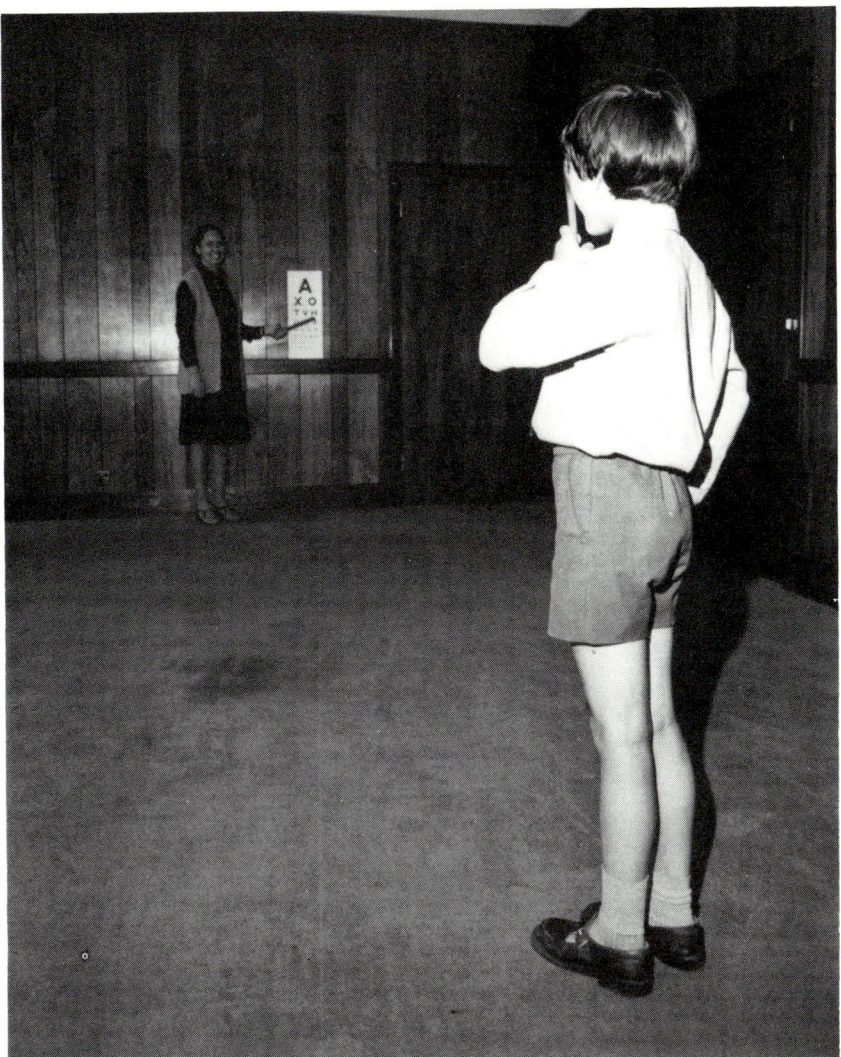

Fig. 9. (a): Distance vision screening at 6 m. Notice the eye-level chart. A second person to help with testing is needed for nursery and infant classes.

removed. Stand the child the correct distance from the chart as illustrated (Fig. 9a). To prevent the child memorizing the letters each line should be read from left to right with one eye and right to left with the other.

The number of the lowest line to be completely read is the one indicating the

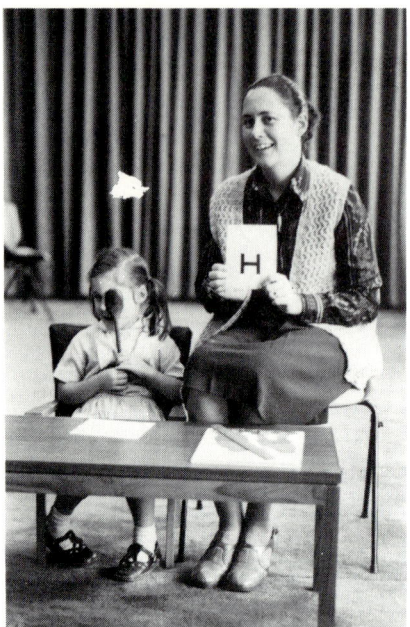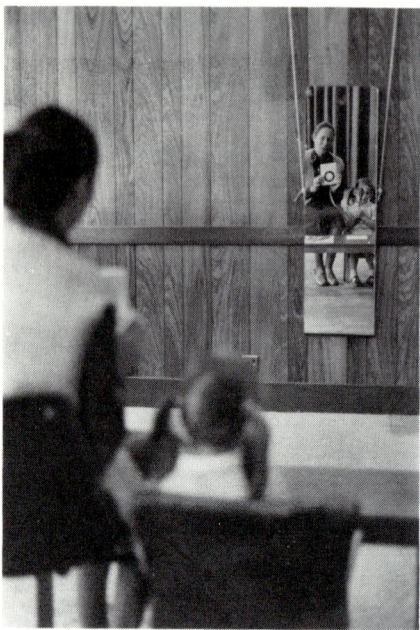

Fig. 9. (b): Testing using a mirror. A key card or plastic letters are provided if child is unable to read.

quality of vision. The result of the test is written as a fraction, for example R 6/60, L 6/6, the first figure indicating the distance at which the child was tested (6 m) and the second the lowest line read. Any child with 6/9 vision, or worse, in one or both eyes should be referred to the school medical officer.

Sometimes the room is too small to conduct the test satisfactorily. Also, it is extremely difficult to keep the attention of a young child at a distance of 6 m unless a second adult is available to help. Consequently, half-sized letter cards may be used at a distance of 3 m, or if the children are not familiar with the names of all the letters, the *mirror test* (Fig. 9b) may be used. This enables the examiner to sit beside the child and control his attention. Reversed letter cards are held slightly above the child's head and reflected in the mirror (at a distance of 3 m). The child may read or use a key card or plastic letters to indicate which letter he sees in the mirror.

Near vision The child is asked to read a sheet of printed letters each line of which is graded in size and marked with a number. This is known as the 'N' scale and the number of the smallest line read by the child is recorded together with the distance at which the child held the card.

Colour-vision This should also be tested in the first year at school so that the teacher may modify teaching methods to suit any child who is colour defective. Abnormalities of colour vision are more common in boys than girls; indeed one can anticipate finding about 6% of boys defective. Any nurse administering this test should ensure that she herself is not colour-blind.

The Ishihara colour vision test is usually used. This is a book of coloured plates made up of dots from which certain letters or figures emerge if the child has perfect colour vision and others emerge if not. The coloured plates spoil easily and must be kept away from sun-light. A paint brush may be used by small children to trace the figures seen so that the plates are not altered by finger marks. Good day-light is also needed as electric light distorts the shades. The instruction book recommends that a varied selection of plates are offered for the test so that the children cannot cheat by memorizing.

Any defect found by any of the tests should be referred to the school doctor who will decide whether the child should be referred to a consultant.

Follow-up

Parental consent to refer the child is required as usual and if the parent is absent during the test, a home visit may need to be made. Once consent has been received, the school doctor will refer the child to the children's eye clinic. Failure to attend the vision clinic should be followed up by discussion with the parents and appropriate arrangements made to facilitate attendance at the next appointment. The child who has had the advantages of treatment explained can often influence the parents; also, teachers may be willing to include this in their teaching.

The child will be seen by the ophthalmologist who will diagnose and prescribe treatment. This may be carried out by the orthoptist or if glasses are prescribed they will be fitted by the ophthalmic or dispensing optician. The school doctor and nurse should know what has been recommended and should see that the teacher is fully aware of the implications of any loss of sight and of the reasons why glasses have been prescribed. For example for treatment of squint, where the teacher may think the uncovered eye is the sound one, it may not be realized that the object of the treatment is to exercise the uncovered eye, the vision of which may be considerably impaired. Children attending school may, if necessary, have two pairs of glasses prescribed free of charge (providing NHS frames are chosen); one to keep in school and one at home or in reserve. Glasses kept in school need to be carefully marked with the child's name to avoid mistakes and muddle. Replacement and repair, applied for on DHSS Form GOS2R, is also free to school children except for safety lenses where the excess cost in comparison with ordinary lenses is borne by the parents.

Children can usually be persuaded to wear glasses when care is taken to give adequate explanation and to ensure that the spectacles fit well, are comfortable and improve the vision (strabismus sometimes being the exception and therefore more difficult to treat). Problems such as teasing by other children are better discussed honestly with the child rather than dismissed. The child should know why the glasses have been prescribed and understand how to clean and care for them. The positive aspects can be emphasized using popular television and sports stars and the like as examples. Support of parents and teachers should be enlisted.

At one time it was thought that children with poor vision should not take part in sports as their sight might be adversely affected by blows or knocks. The general opinion now is that where possible, children should be encouraged to participate and compete in physical activities. There are certain exceptions, notably high myopias at risk of pathological retinal changes and therefore it is obviously wise to have the consultant's advice on each individual child.

Where glasses are worn for sports, they should be splinter-proof, and have toughened or plastic lenses. These are only available through the NHS on clinical grounds for severe handicaps, such as spastics who potentially could be harmed by ordinary lenses. This is unfortunate as ordinary spectacles can easily be smashed in rough games and splinters damage the eyes, thus precluding many children from such sports. The DHSS is now considering this problem. Contact lenses may also be prescribed in certain cases.

The classroom and school lighting should be good. The decor is also important; plain pale matt colours reflect the light best and are the least disturbing to the eyes. Children with a visual handicap who need to have their books close to the eyes should be provided with suitably designed desks or lecterns to prevent them stooping, and the physical education teacher will wish to assist these children with their posture.

Metal reflector Angle-poise lights are best for desk use and should reflect the light onto the child's work without causing shadow or glare.

Another point to remember is that children's sight may be considerably damaged by watching solar eclipses without special eye protection and in these days of practical project work teachers should be warned of this if an eclipse is pending.

Visual Handicap

Any treatment prescribed, either spectacles or contact lenses aims to correct the vision to normal or near normal. However, this is not always possible and some children may be able to see very little indeed even with very powerful visual aids. When, following correction, the sight is only 6/24 to 3/60, a child is said to be moderately visually handicapped; 3/60 and less is severely visually handicapped, although considerations such as ability to use the limited sight and to cope generally will affect such a classification. There are certain advantages in actually being registered as handicapped in that a child will be eligible to be provided with expensive equipment and educational help; also other financial and social assistance will be available to the family.

Assessment for education There should be a team approach including the school medical officer, ophthalmologist, educational psychologist, a teacher for the visually handicapped and the parents, for assessment for education. Placement of the child will vary according to the degree of handicap, the home circumstances, availability of transport, special educational facilities available and the wishes of the parents. The choice of education may be any of the variations between ordinary school with a specialist peripatetic teacher for the visually handicapped to a residential school. As with other handicaps, due consideration must be given to preserving links with the parents and advising them. There should be regular contact with the ophthalmologist and the child health staff. Genetic counselling should also be available for parents and the teenage handicapped child. There also needs to be continual assessment as some of the children may be able to return to ordinary school following a period of specialized help.

Methods of education The aims of education are to teach the child to be as independent as possible and to adjust happily and make the most of life. Blind children have to be taught by non-visual methods such as Braille (Fig. 10) and radio and tape recordings. Partially-sighted children have more scope in that specially large print reading materials may be used as well as audio-visual equipment and closed circuit television. Many of the children may also be supplied with a variety of low vision aids such as telescopic spectacles and magnifiers (Fig. 11).

The 1944 Education Act for the first time defined the partially-sighted as a separate category of handicap from blind and since then their education has taken place in separate establishments. However, there is a growing body of feeling that more flexible arrangements enabling some sharing of classes would be more beneficial.

Employment and further education Planning for future employment needs to begin early and the matter brought to the attention of the careers officer. Children whose vision cannot be corrected to normal will be unable to consider jobs where high visual acuity is demanded. A colour-blind person should not undertake work requiring action on colour signals such as shipping, railways or civil aviation or where colour appreciation is required as in electronics or textile dyeing.

Further educational and vocational training of blind or partially-sighted children is provided through the Royal Normal College, Royal National Institute for the Blind and government training centres. Courses in commerce, piano tuning, telephony and machine operation are available. Grants are available through the local education authority, and, in certain circumstances, the Department of Employment and the Royal National Institute for the Blind may also contribute, as extra equipment such as Braillers, typewriters and tape recorders increase the expense considerably.

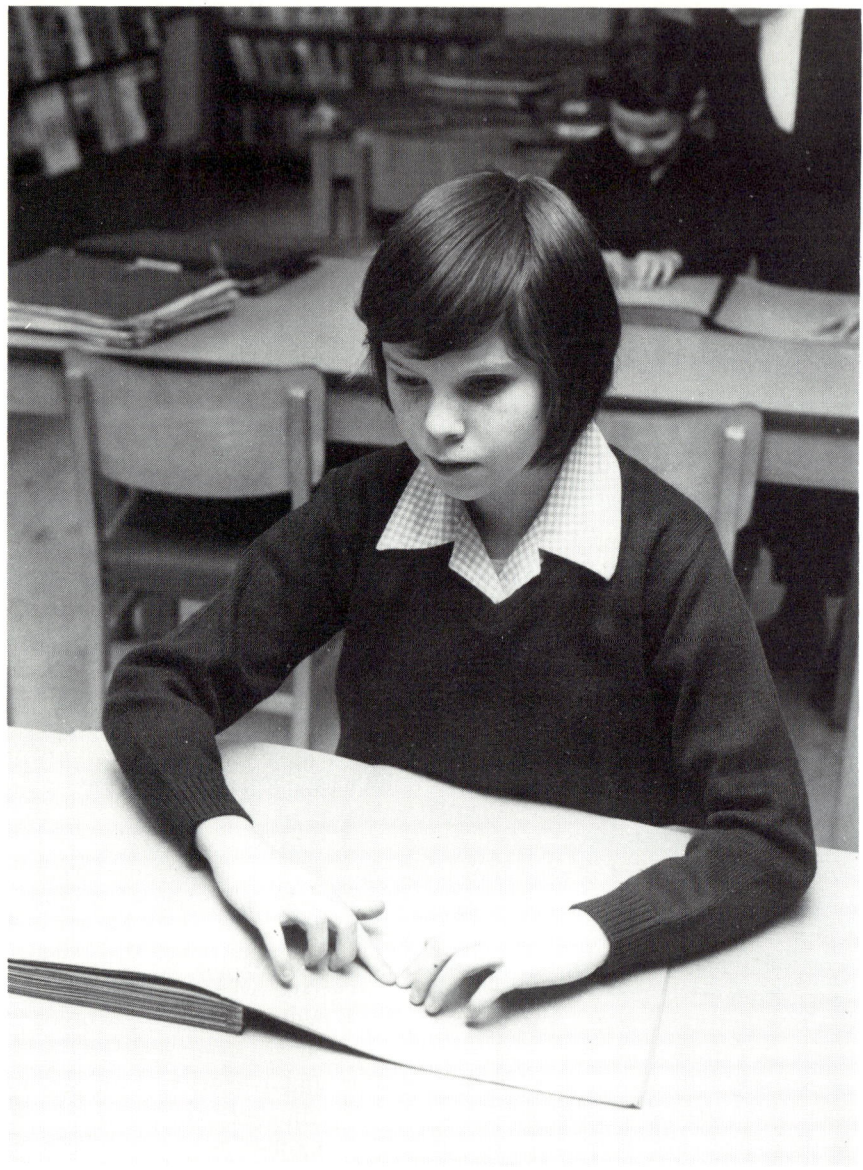

Fig. 10. Learning to read Braille. (Central Office of Information)

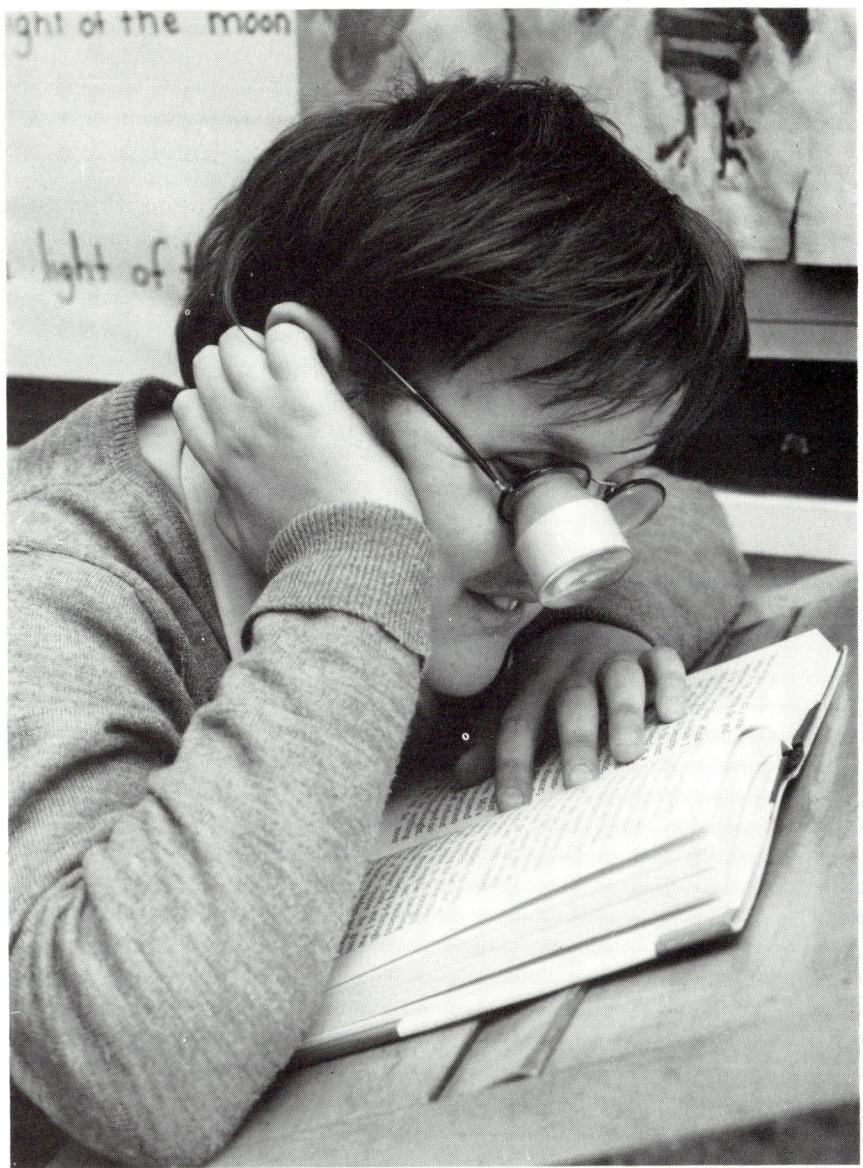

Fig. 11. A partially-sighted child using a low vision aid. The position of the lectern raises the angle of the book and prevents stooping and poor posture. (Central Office of Information)

REFERENCES

1. Trevor Roper, P. (1970) *The World Through Blunted Sight*. London: Thames & Hudson.

FURTHER READING

Eyes Right (1972) London: Consumer Association.

Gramet, C. (1963) *Light and Sight*. London: Abelard-Schuman.

Ingram, T. T. S. (1963) The Association of Speech Retardation and Educational Difficulties. *Proceedings of Royal College of Medicine*, pp. 56, 199–203.

Ishihara, S. *The Series of Plates Designed as a Test for Colour Blindness*. London: H. K. Lewis.

Partially-sighted Children (1972) A summary of their needs and existing provisions. London: National Association for the Education of the Partially-sighted.

Sheridan, M. D. *Manual for the Stycar Vision Test*. London: National Foundation for Education Research in England and Wales.

Smith, H. V. & James, F. E. (1968) *Eyes and Education*. London: Heinemann Medical.

Vernon Report (1968) *The Education of the Visually Handicapped*. London: Department of Education and Science, HMSO.

CHILDREN'S BOOKS

Non-fiction

Elgin, K. (1970) *The Eye*. London: Watts. Primary level.

Nicolls, A. (1975) *Sight*. London: Studio Vista. Primary level.

Shoesmith, K. (1973) *Look and See*. London: Burke. Primary level.

Fiction

Bawden, N. (1966) *The Witch's Daughter*. London: Gollancz. Janey's blindness means that her other senses are well developed which leads her to solving an exciting mystery. 10+ years.

Smith, J. (1973) *Folk Doll of Sion*. London: Hamish Hamilton. Harriet wears glasses to correct a squint and the glasses make it difficult for her to see. Her desire to possess the doll finally leads her to persevere. 7 + years.

Petersen, P. (1976) *Sally Can't See*. London: Black. Well-illustrated picture-book describing how Sally who is blind copes at home, in school and playing games. 6+ years.

USEFUL ADDRESSES AND INFORMATION

The Royal National Institute for the Blind
224–228 Great Portland Street
London W1N 6AA.
Tel: 01 388 1266.

The Partially-Sighted Society
Exhall Grant School
Wheelright Lane
Coventry CV7 9HP.
Tel: Coventry 87334

Membership is free and open to anyone interested and wanting to contribute. Publishes a variety of low-cost leaflets and booklets obtainable from Mr G. H. Marshall.

The National Association for the Education of the Partially-Sighted
Joseph Clarke School
Vincent Road
Highams Park
London E4 9PP.
Tel: 01 527 8818.
Mr R. J. Crosbie (Hon. Secretary)

The Disabled Living Foundation
24b Kensington High Street
London W14 8NS.
Tel: 01 602 2491.

Has a permanent exhibition of low vision aids and other suitable appliances.

Optical Information Council
Walter House
418–422 Strand
London WC2R 0PB.
Tel: 01 836 2323.

Exists to promote eye care and services available to the public. Produces helpful posters, fact sheets and booklets.

In Touch
(BBC programme each Sunday, on Radio 4 at 5 p.m.)
BBC
Broadcasting House
London W1A 1AA.
Tel: 01 580 4468.

Publishes a quarterly bulletin of aids and services for the blind and partially-sighted available from the BBC.

Discussion Topics

1. You notice several of the children who should be using spectacles are not wearing them. How might you influence these children to use them? If the situation persisted, what would you do?

2. The first-aider reports that Louise frequently complains of headaches. You also notice that she has reached puberty. What might this lead you to suspect and how would you test your suspicions?

3. You notice a child's written work contains many reversed letters. What might you suspect and what action would you take?

4. You read in the newspaper that there is to be a solar eclipse in two weeks' time. Would this information warrant any action in school?

5. A boy who is colour-blind tells you he is hoping to be a train driver. How might you react?

6. The doctor has given permission for a partially-sighted child wearing glasses to take part in all school sports. An irate parent arrives at the medical room pronouncing this to be totally incorrect. How might you deal with the situation?

6
Hearing Screening

To be deaf or even slightly deaf is one of the saddest handicaps because, although most people are sympathetic initially, it is easy to become irritated either by constantly having to raise one's voice or, even worse, by the strain of communicating with someone who cannot hear at all. Surgical operations or even hearing aids are not always the answer and some children can expect to live all their lives in a world of muffled sound or total silence. Unfortunately, the main cause of permanent deafness are defects or damage to the cochlea or the auditory nerve and at present there is no known cure.

A useful experiment in trying to understand the problems facing such a child is to turn the television sound down to a level that cannot be heard properly, or not at all, and then watch the programme. You will find yourself straining to hear and desperately looking for gestures, signs and facial expressions which will indicate what is being said. It is not difficult to see that faced with such a situation from babyhood, early training and use of any aids which will improve the hearing is essential if a child is to grow up to live a satisfactory happy life. For this reason hearing tests are administered at various stages of childhood, the optimum age for the first one being between 7 and 9 months. Often the parents will suspect a child is deaf and they are usually right. The doctor or health visitor will be most likely to suspect a hearing defect in a child from a family with a history of deafness and the mother suspects the baby is deaf, or when a child is late in learning to babble and speak. Where there is a history of maternal rubella or anoxia or jaundice during birth and the neonatal period, the visual and motor pathways may also be affected, resulting in a child with not only a hearing defect but multiple handicaps. As soon as hearing loss is discovered it is investigated and appropriate treatment begins. In the event of permanent hearing loss the parents need immediate specialized help from a qualified teacher of the deaf so that auditory training and language teaching may begin.

Some children only have a slight hearing loss or a temporary reduction in one or both ears for one reason or another. This can often pass unnoticed and the child may be thought to be a slow learner or stupid; indeed, it has been suggested that some 5% of primary school children suffer some degree of deafness. To discover this all children should have an audiometric screening test at school entry and on at least one other occasion before leaving their primary school. Certainly, no child should be considered for special education without being given a hearing test. Any child who has recently had an illness which might result in hearing loss or who is suspected of being deaf by, for example, teacher or parent, should have the test repeated. Screening tests may be carried out either by the school nurse or audiometrician. To explain the circumstances in which problems may occur, it is necessary to re-state the mechanism and anatomy of hearing.

Hearing Mechanism

Moving objects produce vibrations in the air. Some of these are detected by the human ear and pass along the hearing pathway to the brain where they are interpreted. We hear sounds at varying degrees of loudness and pitch and it is possible to hear certain sounds perfectly well and not others. This is very important in speech as every sound we utter has a different degree of loudness and pitch; consequently, a person with severe hearing loss will produce sounds without any intonation and most of us are familiar with the flat monotonous tone of speech produced by some people with hearing impairment. Vowels sound in the lower range of notes and consonants higher; consequently, a person with a hearing loss for higher notes will have a very distorted idea of speech. To have some idea of this, try reading a sentence aloud, leaving out all the consonants.

Damage or obstruction to the external and middle ear structures may cause permanent or temporary loss of hearing known as *conductive* deafness. This usually represents a reduction in the loudness of sounds and can often be cured by medical treatment. Damage to any part of the inner ear or central auditory pathway causes hearing loss known as *sensorineural* or *perceptive deafness*. Conductive hearing loss is a much simpler type of loss which can be overcome by amplification of sound. Perceptive deafness is much more complex in that other attributes of hearing are distorted, for example perception of loudness, and therefore it is much more difficult to compensate.

The Ear

The outer ear This is a narrow tube called the external auditory canal which funnels the sound to the tympanic membrane (or ear drum) which forms a division between the outer and the middle ear (see Fig. 12). Temporary deafness may occur in the following circumstances:

1. Wax may accumulate becoming hard and dry and muffling the sound. Normal hearing will return when the wax is removed.

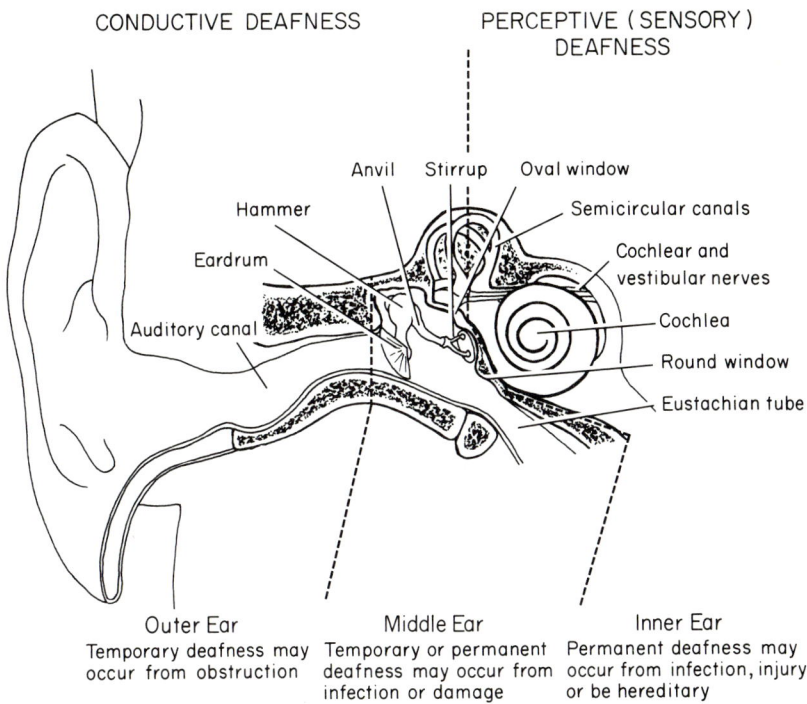

CONDUCTIVE DEAFNESS   PERCEPTIVE (SENSORY) DEAFNESS

Anvil   Stirrup   Oval window

Hammer   Semicircular canals

Eardrum   Cochlear and vestibular nerves

Auditory canal   Cochlea

Round window

Eustachian tube

Outer Ear	Middle Ear	Inner Ear
Temporary deafness may occur from obstruction	Temporary or permanent deafness may occur from infection or damage	Permanent deafness may occur from infection, injury or be hereditary

Fig. 12. The anatomy of the ear indicating possible forms of deafness.

2. Beads, peas, bits of pencil and other objects may be poked into the ear by the child. They should be removed by the doctor as otherwise infection and discharge may result.

The middle ear This is an enclosed space bounded by the tympanic membrane and the oval and round window opening into the inner ear canal. The middle ear contains three small bones, the malleus, incus and stapes (hammer, anvil and stirrup), which are connected to each other and rock backwards and forwards vibrating the sounds through the inner ear. The action in the middle ear is said to increase the force of the sound some fifteen times. Protection against very loud noises is afforded by the inter-tympanic muscles which contract at the impact of a loud sound.

Air pressure is regulated by means of a small passage known as the eustachian tube. This is lined with mucous membrane and runs between the middle ear and the nasopharynx and is generally the means by which infection travels from the throat to the ear.

Otitis media and glue ear are by far the commonest causes of middle ear hearing loss in young school children, mainly because of the high incidence of upper respiratory tract infections in this country.

Otitis media This is an infection of the middle ear generally causing a painful throbbing ear-ache. The infection usually enters via the eustachian tube and is secondary to infections of tonsils or adenoids, heavy colds or obstruction of the nose, respiratory infection, measles or influenza. The child should be referred to the doctor immediately for treatment. Neglected otitis media can result in a perforated ear drum and a persistently discharging ear which may cause varying degrees of hearing loss or even mastoiditis, meningitis or brain abscess.

Glue ear This is an increasingly common condition among children under the age of 12 years. The 'glue' is a mucous fluid which blocks the eustachian tube and can result in temporary or permanent deafness. The cause is uncertain but it is thought in some cases to be the result of partially treated otitis media which removes the earache and symptoms, but not the condition itself. Therefore, it is important to see that courses of antibiotics given for otitis media are completed, following which the ears should be thoroughly re-examined. Glue ear can be diagnosed by otoscopic examination or more recently by tympanometry which is a special test measuring the mobility of the ear drum and the condition of the middle ear.

Inner ear This consists of the cochlea and the semicircular canals and is also known as the labyrinth. The cochlea resembles a snail shell covered in tiny hair cells and its function is to convert sound waves into electrical stimuli which pass along the auditory nerve to the brain where they are interpreted. The semi-circular canals are concerned with balance.

Inner ear hearing loss may result from the following:

1. Hereditary defect or virus infection such as rubella contracted by the mother in early stages of pregnancy, resulting in various degrees of sensorineural deafness.
2. Severe systemic infection, for example meningitis.
3. Injury from severe blow fracturing the bone structure and damaging the cochlea.
4. Constant exposure to excessively loud sound or to sudden very loud noise (gun fire) causes paralysis of the hair cells of the cochlea, resulting in progressive incurable deafness, starting at the higher frequencies and gradually spreading to the lower ones.

Deafness may affect both ears (bilateral) or one ear (unilateral). A child with unilateral deafness has an obvious advantage in having normal hearing in one ear and this is generally adequate for most purposes. However, it does have the effect that one cannot distinguish the direction of sound. This can be dangerous, particularly in traffic, and children with this type of deafness need special instruction in road safety.

General Indications of Possible Deafness

Sometimes the child's mannerisms or conduct in class might lead to a suspicion of hearing loss. Investigations would be warranted should any of the following be noticed.

1. Mispronunciation of words or particular consonants, slipshod speech or a peculiar pitch of voice.
2. Failure to respond when spoken to unless facing the speaker.
3. Inaccurate spelling and reproduction of dictation, incompatible with the standard of work on other occasions.
4. Tendency to listen with head turned to one side.
5. Not understanding what is being said; either speaking at the same time, giving irrelevant answers, or asking for questions to be repeated.
6. Complaints of noises, ringing or buzzing in the ears or head.
7. Constant colds, mouth breathing, or upper respiratory tract infections.
8. Starts demonstrating emotional problems, becoming very naughty, aloof or suspicious, or adopting a careless indifferent attitude.

All 'non-communicating' children are not necessarily deaf although every child with communication problems should have a screening test to exclude deafness as a cause. Difficulties with language and speech may also be the result of perceptual problems, autism or mental retardation.

Screening Screening for hearing impairment may be done by a variety of tests depending on the age of the child. In infants these may be based on behavioural observation. In young children various types of speech tests may be used and older children generally respond to screen audiometric tests.

Tests for hearing speech sounds There are a great variety of speech tests. However, in school, the child is usually asked to repeat certain words or sentences specially formulated to test hearing for vowels (low frequency) and consonants (high frequency). The tester stands 3 m from a young child (under seven years) or 5 m from an older child. These tests are of little use with children who have a poor vocabulary or know very little English.

Audiometer screening test An audiometer is used to test hearing for pure tones and the result is recorded on an audiogram chart. The volume or loudness of the sounds heard is measured in units (decibels) ranging from −10 or 0 to 120 and charted on the vertical column of the audiogram. The frequency ranges from 125 to 8000 cycles per second and is shown on the horizontal line of the chart marked Hz (Hertz being the name of the scientist who first named and fixed the measurement). The audiogram gives a clear indication of the type and degree of hearing loss, for example a loss on the low frequencies is likely to be conductive while the higher frequencies can indicate perceptive deafness (Fig. 13) although this will need to be confirmed by comparison between air and bone conduction tests.

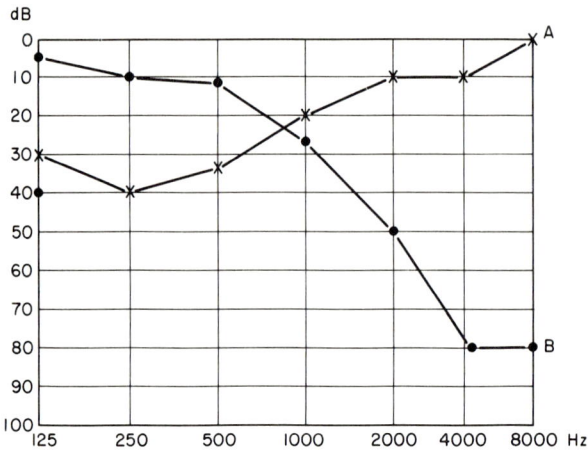

Fig. 13. A pure tone audiogram illustrating conductive and perceptive deafness. A: hearing loss on low tones typical of conductive deafness. B: high frequency hearing loss typical of perceptive deafness

There are, of course, very sophisticated audiometers used at audiology centres. However, the audiometer used in school is a simple model and the screen test is only designed to identify children needing more accurate investigation. The equipment, as it is being moved from school to school, is likely to be damaged and therefore needs regular frequent servicing to ensure that the readings are accurate.

To conduct a screening test conditions of reasonable quiet are needed. The head teacher should be asked to allocate as quiet a room as possible. However, if this presents difficulties, alternatives need to be considered. Head-sets designed to exclude as much noise as possible are available or the children could attend the local clinic or health centre with a sound-proofed room. Some authorities provide suitably designed mobile units which can be parked in the school grounds.

The test is totally dependent on the child indicating each time a sound is heard, and a shy, frightened or belligerent child may hear perfectly well but fail to respond. Therefore, it is essential that time is spent, particularly with young children, in gaining co-operation by explaining and demonstrating the procedure, allowing the children to handle the head-sets and hear the sounds the equipment makes. Such explanations are usually made to groups of five to ten children, five being the maximum number of young children that may easily be controlled. The youngest are usually given some bricks or pegs to place in a box when a sound is heard, while older children usually indicate by raising a hand. The ear-phones are carefully placed in position only when it is felt that the child fully understands the procedure. Each ear is tested separately and it is wise to make a habit of always starting with the left ear so that any muddle in charting is avoided. The volume is then set at 20 decibels which it has been agreed represents the level at which speech can be heard in normal school conditions. In particularly difficult conditions it may be raised to 25 decibels on the lower frequencies only. The frequencies of 250, 500, 1000, 2000, 4000 and 8000 are then presented, starting at 1000 followed by the frequencies above and below. The time intervals between each sound should be varied so that the child does not cheat by anticipating a regular pattern. For the same reason care needs to be taken to see that the nurse is not observed moving the dials of the machine (Fig. 14). Failure to respond to any frequency may only be

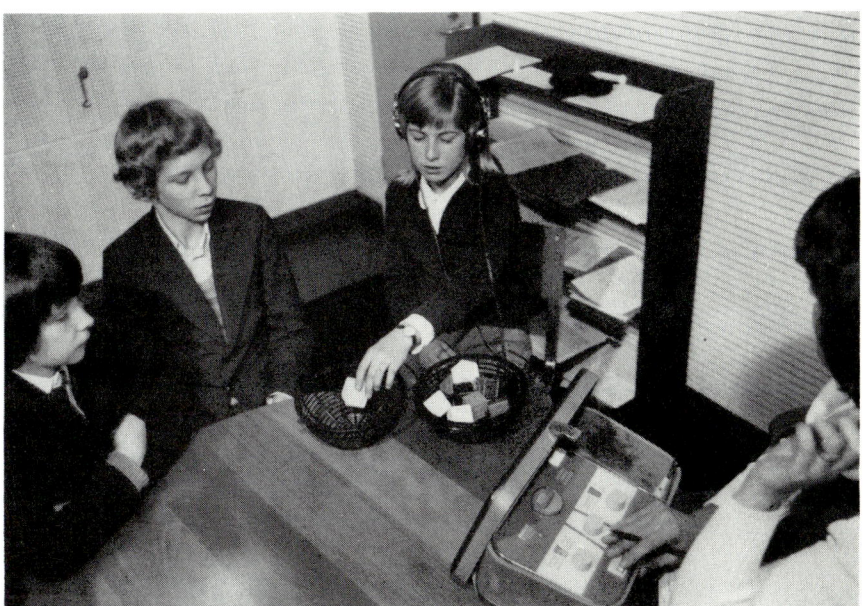

Fig. 14. Conducting a 'sweep' test. (Camera Talks Ltd)

a temporary occurrence, for example as a result of a head cold, in which case the test should be repeated in two weeks. To avoid mistakes, a doubtful response should always be regarded as a failure. A second failure indicates the need for a full threshold screen test. Tests are not charted on an audiogram but a note should be made in the medical record indicating that the test was carried out and whether the child passed or failed.

A full threshold test in which the frequencies 250 to 8000 are presented at reducing 10 decibel steps from 60 to 0 is carried out in a sound-proofed audiometric room. The results are recorded on an audiogram and entered in the medical record. A child who fails to respond to any frequency on this test should be referred by the doctor to the audiologist who will conduct a range of pure-tone, air and bone conduction, and speech tests. The difficulty in audiometry is the dependence on the co-operation of the child and at present a considerable amount of work is being done to develop tests which record physiological responses, irrespective of participation.

The class-teacher should be informed by the nurse if there is any suspicion of hearing loss so that, without drawing attention to the matter, the child can sit near to the teacher with the best ear in the direction of the teacher's or other children's voices if discussion is taking place.

Comprehensive Assessment

Once the cause of the deafness is known treatment may be instituted. Where no medical or surgical treatment can repair the damage, hearing aids may be needed so that the child can make full use of any residual hearing. Consideration must be given to placing the child in the most suitable school

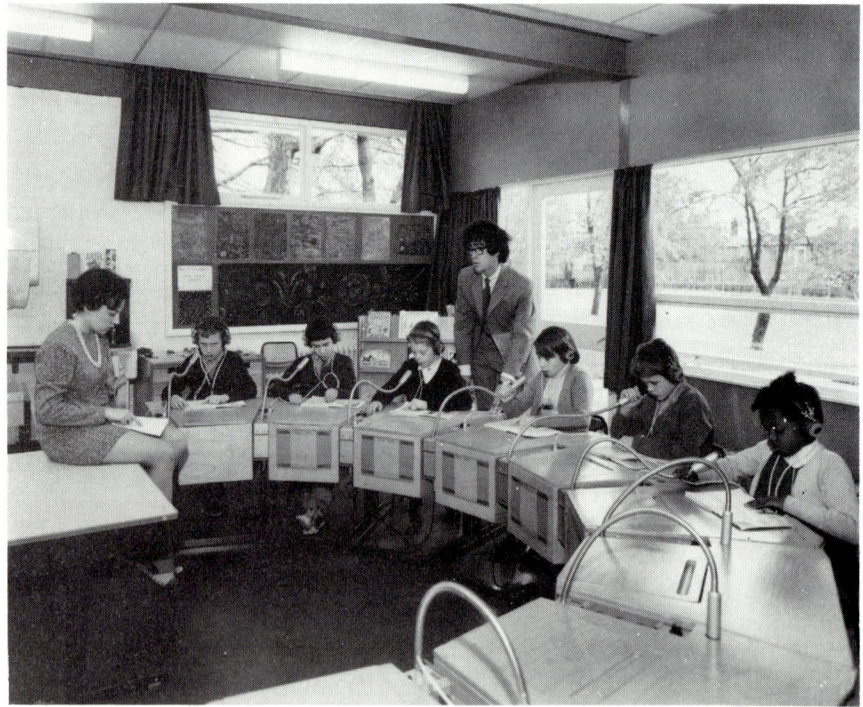

Fig. 15. *Pupils wearing individually adjusted earphones listen to the teacher who uses a microphone. (John Sani)*

and special day and residential facilities are available together with special units attached to ordinary schools. These units are equipped for sound amplification and each child may have individually adjusted ear-phones (Fig. 15). Rooms fitted with loop induction coils facilitate movement around the class-room while still picking up the sounds.

School placement should be planned in consultation with the parents, the audiological physician, speech therapist, teacher for the deaf, child psychiatrist, educational psychologist and the social worker. Should the child be thought to require special educational facilities, the procedure for obtaining this should be set in motion (see p. 104). Parents need to be fully involved and helped to understand the child's limitations and the best methods of coping and encouraging the child. Genetic counselling should also be available to them in the event of their planning to have another child and later to their handicapped adolescent, if the deafness is hereditary.

The kind of school placement required will be influenced (as are all handicaps) by the degree of handicap and the range of facilities available, the intelligence and ability of the child, previous experience of speech and language if the deafness is acquired, and the amount of parental support and interest which he is likely to receive.

Table 1 represents a very broad guide to some of the possibilities.

Methods of Education

The greater the degree of hearing loss the more difficult it is to teach the child and the more skill, patience and effort required. The methods adopted will vary according to the amount of speech and language the child already has, the child with an acquired loss of hearing having had the considerable advantage of experiencing normal speech and conversation. Although attempts to teach the profoundly deaf have been made since the sixteenth century, recent surveys indicate that the majority of deaf children even today are still far behind in reading, speech and comprehension of language, one survey estimating a reading age of 8 years for most 16-year-olds. Intonation of voice is necessary for speech to be easily understood but is very difficult to demonstrate to the deaf child and it is estimated that over half of all deaf children still have unintelligible speech. A variety of visual and electronic aids are being used and developed to improve the child's ability to articulate and produce intelligible speech.

Experts are divided in their views on the best methods of teaching. Special units for the deaf and partially-hearing are equipped to amplify sound and use group hearing aids (as mentioned on p. 78, Fig. 15). Lip-reading and sign-language were at one time discouraged but they are now thought to help in acquiring vocabulary and language and are being widely taught, the movements of sound being copied and the vibrations learned by touching the teacher's face as she speaks (Fig. 16). Developments in audiometry techniques

Table 1.   The education of children with various degrees of hearing loss

Everyday sounds	Decibels	Degree of loss	Effects	Education
Hearing threshold	0			
Rustle of a leaf	10	Mild loss	May have minor effect on speech and language	Attend ordinary school; teacher should be alerted and child sit with ear with most hearing in direction of sound and able to watch whoever is speaking
	20	Mild loss		
Whisper	30	Mild loss		
	40	Partial loss	Difficulty in hearing ordinary speech; may require hearing-aid	May attend ordinary school with support from peripatetic teacher or partially-hearing unit attached to ordinary school
	50	Partial loss		
Ordinary conversation	60	Partial loss		
Private car Television	70	Severe loss	Fails to hear a conversation and understand it; needs support and training at home using hearing-aid	Partially-hearing unit attached to ordinary school or day or residential partially-hearing school
Crying child	80	Severe loss		
Loud drum at 1 m, underground train	90	Severe loss		
Heavy lorry	100	Profound loss	May hear some sounds when using powerful hearing-aid; relies on other forms of communication; needs intensive support in the home	Day or residential school for the deaf
Pneumatic drill at close range	110	Profound loss		

and production of more sensitive hearing aids have been speedily advancing since the 1940s and should benefit more children although once prescribed, unless they are actually used, they cannot hope to be effective.

Use of hearing aid All teaching staff and any adult who has contact with a deaf or partially-hearing child using a hearing aid should understand the conditions which will either reduce the effectiveness of the hearing aid or render it useless. Every effort should be made to see that optimum use of a hearing aid is achieved. Hearing aids have developed considerably in recent years and not only can they amplify sound but certain frequencies can be selected for greater amplification than others. A child who has been successfully fitted with a

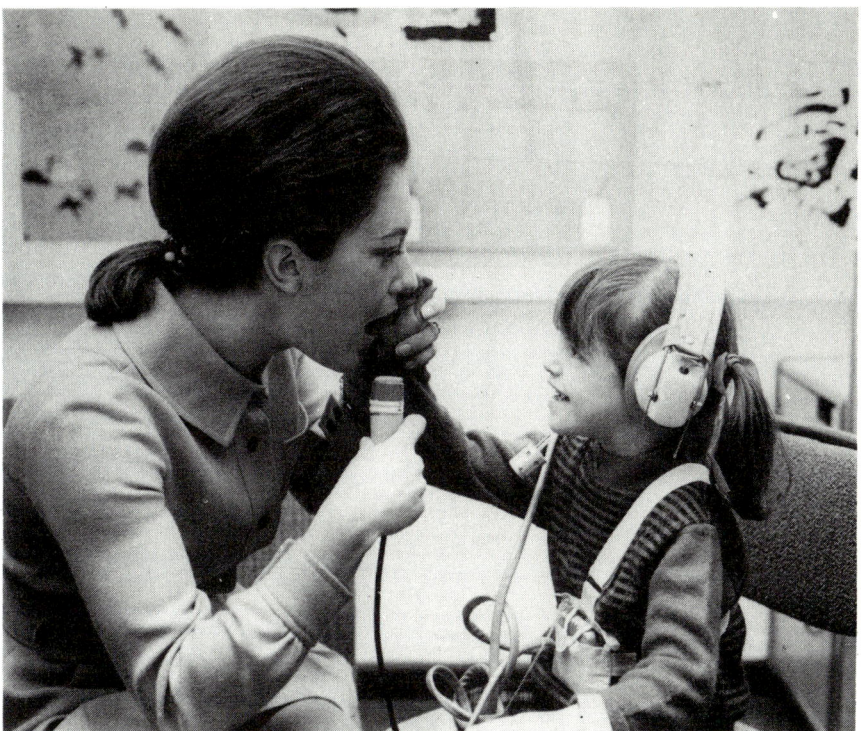

Fig. 16. Feeling the movements of sound and seeing the shape each one makes. (Central Press)

properly selected aid will wear it and use it continually because of the obvious benefit. They will also report any fault immediately and will usually keep the aid switched well on rather than turned down or off. A child who complains or is distressed by the aid has usually been incorrectly fitted or supplied with an unsuitable model.

There are a variety of aids available, some designed and supplied under the NHS and some designed by commercial firms. The choice will depend on the type of hearing loss and the age and circumstances of the child. The audiology physician will instruct the child and the parents in the use of the aid. However, a nurse working in a special school for deaf or partially-hearing children should be in regular contact with the audiology unit and be fully familiar with the aids supplied to individual children. Body-worn aids are those most frequently used by school children and in general the microphone should face outwards and occlusion from limbs or garments should be avoided. It should be tested daily to see that it is in working order and ear moulds should be clean and free of wax. These need to be re-fitted regularly while the child is growing as ill-fitting moulds will cause whistling and buzzing noises. Any of these complaints should be immediately reported to the audiologist. Generally, a period of about six months is required following the initial fitting for the child to become fully familiar with its use and for assessment to be made as to the benefit for the child. A number of useful information booklets are published by the DHSS and various voluntary organizations such as the Royal National Institute for the Deaf.

Social services Families with a child known to have permanent hearing loss, whether partial or severe, are likely to need a good deal of practical, material and moral support to enable them to help the child. Some social services have specialist social workers for the deaf or they enlist the support of specialist social workers from voluntary organizations. Volunteer support is also growing and since 1974 the National Deaf Children's Society have organized training for parents of older deaf children to assist teachers of the deaf, usually in their work with families by occupying and caring for other children while the teacher and parent are involved with the deaf child, or by giving the mother the moral support of similar past experience.

Future career As with other handicaps, the careers officer needs to be involved at an early stage. Unfortunately, there are still relatively few vocational training courses and facilites for further education are limited. Consequently, many able partially-hearing adolescents find themselves in menial undemanding jobs which lead to frustration and emotional difficulties.

Prevention Planning ahead to avoid deafness in the next generation is an equally important aspect of school health work. Rubella vaccination programmes in secondary schools are designed to minimize the risks of virus infection in early pregnancy causing blindness and deafness in the newborn. Consequently, due care needs to be given to promote this among adolescent girls and to see that female teachers have also been protected and are themselves reminded of the consequences should rubella be diagnosed among the children. Early attention to ear-aches and discharges prevents damage from chronic conditions and it is wise to have the doctor re-examine the ear-drum following a course of anti-biotics. This avoids chronic low grade infections; indeed, it would seem sensible for nurses working in schools to undertake this. Good school policies for infectious diseases and accident prevention go some way to avoiding hearing loss caused by unnecessary infection or accident.

Hearing is sometimes affected by certain antibiotics and occasionally by aspirin. It is therefore important that parents are aware of the need to draw a new doctor's attention to the hearing defect if antibiotics are being prescribed for acute infections.

The effects of noise, not only on hearing, but on health generally, are thought by many to be one of the serious problems of the future. Therefore, it is appropriate here to mention some aspects in relation to the school. The level of noise in the building generally can affect learning in that attention may be distracted from the teacher and concentration will wane if a child cannot hear what is being said properly. School acoustic design and siting of rooms for various activities takes this into account. Sound also has an emotional and psychological effect, for example soft music can calm us, and loud pop music can send adolescent girls into hysteria. Absence of sound may cause fear, while repetitive incessant sound, such as dripping taps, can cause irritation and anger or if taken to extremes, as practised in torture chambers, it may result in mental disorder. Studies of high levels of noise in industry have shown physiological changes occurring in heart rhythms and decreased blood circulation while concentration and memory may be affected to a degree that seriously reduces work output.

The power of sound in the production of heat and energy is being continually researched. Bomb blasts and rifle fire at close range can cause permanent hearing damage but more subtle risks emerge as uses for ultrasonic (above the level of human hearing) and infrasonic (below the level of human hearing) sounds are being developed in all walks of life, not least the medical profession itself. It is now possible to destroy and damage not only the hearing mechanism but many other body cells and tissues without hearing anything.

The harmful effects of noise should be an in-built part of teaching in practical work departments and health education programmes. Children should learn to automatically protect their hearing while using equipment which produces high noise levels. This is good training and preparation for jobs in industry.

FURTHER READING

Ballantyne, J. (1977) *Deafness*, 3rd ed. Harlow, Essex: Churchill Livingstone.

Chedd, G. (1970) *Sound—Its Uses and Abuses in Today's Technology*. London: Aldus Books.

In Defence of Hearing (1976) P.O. Box 56, 47 Bell Street, Henley on Thames, Oxon.: Bilson International.

DHSS Booklet HA1 (1975) *General Guidance to Hearing-aid Users*. London: HMSO.

Guidelines in Environmental Designs in Educational Buildings. (1974) London: Architects and Building Branch, DES.

National College of the Deaf and Society of Teachers of the Deaf (Joint Committee Report) (1976) *The Hearing-impaired Child in your Class*. London: Royal National Institute for the Deaf.

Kershaw, J. D. (1973) The Audiology Revolution. *Public Health*, pp. 87, 99–105.

Rawson Report (1973) *Deafness—Report of a Departmental Inquiry into the Promotion of Research*. London: DHSS Reports on Health and Social Subjects, HMSO.

Rutter, M. & Martin, J. A. M. (1972) (eds) *The Child with Delayed Speech*. London: Heinemann Medical.

Watson, T. J. (1967) *The Education of Hearing-handicapped Children*. London: University Press.

CHILDREN'S BOOKS

Non-fiction

Elgin, K. (1973) *Listen and Hear*. London: Burke. Use Your Senses Series, primary very elementary.

Nicholls, A. (1975) *Hearing*. London: Studio Vista. Primary level.

Shoesmith, K. (1973) *Listen and Hear* London: Burke. Primary level, very elementary.

Fiction

Peter, D. (1976) *Claire and Emma*. London: Black. Beautiful picture book describing how Claire and Emma both wear hearing-aids, learn to lip-read and speak and cope with life generally. Clair attends a special school. Primary level.

Robinson, V. (1965) *David in Silence*. London: André Deutsch. David is deaf and has difficulty making friends. On an adventure in a canal tunnel, David is the only one who is not frightened because he is used to silence. 10+ years.

Spence, E. (1972) *Nothing Place*. Oxford: University Press. Glen is partially deaf and will not wear his hearing aid. He hides his deafness at his new school which results in mis-understandings. Glen gradually comes to terms with his disability. 10+ years.

USEFUL ADDRESSES AND INFORMATION

Deaf, Blind and Rubella Children's Society
164 Cromwell Road
Coventry CB4 8AH.
Tel: 0203 (Coventry) 462579.

Organizes conferences and produces literature and films, concerning the plight of children handicapped as a result of rubella. Also produces promotional material aimed at increasing up-take of rubella vaccination in schoolgirls.

National Deaf Children's Society
31 Gloucester Place
London W1H 4EA.
Tel: 01 486 3251.

Publishes extremely helpful information, including a quarterly magazine *Talk* devoted to the interests of the deaf child.

The Royal National Institute for the Deaf
105 Gower Street
London WC1.
Tel: 01 387 8033.

Discussion Topics

1. What is the most effective action the school nurse can take to prevent deafness in the future?

2. A child who has recently had several bouts of coughs and colds seems to have lost interest in class work. The teacher complains he does not pay attention and talks to other children while she is addressing the class. What might you suspect and what action would you take?

3. A child who uses a hearing aid is continually switching it off. What might you suspect and what action would be needed?

4. Consider ways in which a peripatetic teacher for the deaf might be of assistance to you in your work and vice versa.

5. You are conducting an audiometric screening of the children and are doubtful about some of the responses. What would you do?

6. Consider any special help or attention which might be given to a partially-hearing child in an ordinary school.

7
Mental Health

All experiences of life have emotional implications for the individuals concerned. Children's emotional responses vary at each age level and the capacity to cope with the pressures of living, learning and growing up differs from child to child. Learning to manage successfully one's own personal difficulties is part of the preparation for becoming a well-adjusted and healthy adult, and achieving this is an important responsibility of the school's educational aims. The school should not compound a child's problems by reinforcing them but should rather seek to support the child and his family so that his learning and general development can progress satisfactorily. Sometimes these problems may only need a little understanding and help from the teacher or the social worker, but they may require medical and/or psychiatric referral, or need a wide range of team expertise. Pressures on a child may be many and diverse, ranging from problems in the home, the surrounding community or indeed the school. Children may not get on well with their teachers or fellow pupils or there may be friction in the adult school community generating a disturbed and troubled atmosphere. Alternatively, the fault may lie either in the child himself or in his inability to compete successfully with his classmates. Equally, exceptionally able children subjected to lessons that fail to stretch their capabilities and intelligence may also demonstrate behaviour disturbances.

The mental health problems arising in schools are now far greater than those of a physical nature (see p. 20) although the incidence in schools will vary considerably. They seem to be greater in urban rather than rural areas and somewhat higher in boys than girls, depending on the type of disorder; for example conduct disorders are more common in boys, neurotic cases are slightly more common among girls. In addition the understanding of the staff and the ability to identify and treat will affect the incidence in a district.

The school nurse has a role to play in conjunction with the rest of the staff to prevent, recognize and help in the management of these problems. To do this she needs to be aware of the kind of problems likely to be encountered, the children most likely to be affected and the school system for dealing with them. She also needs to be aware of the activities of school generally, including the work displayed by children and she needs to associate it with her own know-ledge of each child. Children's behaviour may be observed under a variety of circumstances and may be totally different in the classroom, playground or the home. The school nurse attends the school more regularly and sees the children more frequently than the doctor, and consequently her observations will be important in drawing attention to particular children.

Children's disturbances are a lot less clearly defined than adults and child psychiatrists are seeking to group and classify them so that they may be better understood. A World Health Organization seminar in 1969 produced a classification on three scales. However, in the context of this book, it is sufficient to list the broad groupings as follows:

1. Antisocial and conduct disorders (truancy, lying, stealing, destructive behaviour, violence, petty theft).
2. Neurotic disorders (anxiety and phobias, school refusal, depression, obessional neurosis, hysterics); children often show a mixed pattern of both antisocial and neurotic behaviour.
3. Specific delays and disorders (poor speech and language, slow learning, clumsiness, tics, toilet problems, enuresis, encopresis, eating and sleeping difficulties).
4. Psychosis.

The majority of normal children will demonstrate behaviour disturbances at one time or another and they only become a cause for serious concern when they are persistent and start to interfere with the child's learning and development. We also know that these disturbances are more likely to arise and be of a serious nature in certain types of children, namely:

1. Children who have spent periods of time in foster-care or separated from the home during early childhood.
2. Children who have had repeated hospital admissions before the age of five years.
3. Handicapped children, particularly severely mentally handicapped and those with epilepsy and conditions involving brain pathology.
4. Children of families with long-standing social, marital or health problems.

Group 1. Antisocial and Conduct Disorders

These are by far the most common occurrences and in recent years the increasing number of children committing quite serious crimes has become a problem of national concern. All children are naughty from time to time and this is perfectly normal. Indeed, it would be surprising and suspicious to find a child who is always good. However, a child who is persistently disruptive, disobedient and aggressive warrants serious investigation into the possible cause. This may be accompanied by or progress to lying, stealing and violence which in adolescence is often associated with smoking, drinking and drug-taking. Some youngsters eventually resort to shop-lifting, petty theft, house-breaking and vandalism. A sizeable proportion of adults convicted of criminal behaviour have a history of this pattern of behaviour in childhood and adolescence.

This kind of behaviour is frequently found in children who are backward in reading. To be constantly bottom of the class and a failure at everything must be a devastating experience, comparable to being continually subjected to a foreign language of which one understands practically nothing. Under such circumstances it is not difficult to understand the enticing prospect of establishing oneself as the class nuisance, admired by one's peers for daring behaviour.

Truancy, i.e. non-attendance at school without the consent of parents or school staff, is often a sign that things are going very wrong and children are seeking to escape continual school failure. Absences from school need immediate investigation by the education welfare officer to establish the reason. Serious consideration must then be given by teachers, social workers, and doctors alike as to how the individual problem may be tackled.

Group 2. Neurotic Disorders

Anxiety is also a normal part of life. It is usual to be anxious about a forth-coming examination or an interview, and to some degree we need this reaction to spur us on to prepare properly for success. Most adults know that this kind of stress can cause physical pain and have experienced the tight restricted throat which often accompanies grief, diarrhoea before an important event, the empty stomach feeling of missing a loved one, but children often do not connect the cause and effect and frequently complain of pains and aches associated with the next lesson, examinations, or the like. Someone must sit down to explain this or discover if the complaint has a more serious origin. Anxiety which is exaggerated to a degree that produces constant physical or behavioural disturbance, interfering with a child's daily life is abnormal. In childhood most neurotic behaviour disappears after a time whether or not it is treated. However, sometimes it persists into adult life but it is extremely difficult to identify whether or not it is likely to be long-term.

Anxiety state This is very common, particularly among children who seem unable to concentrate in class. Discussion with parents usually reveals that the child is having difficulty in sleeping or walks in his sleep or has nightmares. Sometimes the child is afraid in the dark or he is terrified of hobgoblins or he may be scared of ordinary everyday activities such as going to school. Fear may be manifested physically by diarrhoea, vomiting, wetting or persistent headaches.

School refusal This is absence from school because of the sudden onset of illness just before it is time for school. This may be very real in terms of vomiting, diarrhoea, pains in the tummy or headache. It usually disappears during the day and is totally absent at weekends or during the school holiday. It is most frequent among children who are alone a lot or who withdraw from activities with other children. The parents of these children are often over-protective and fussy. Children with a true irrational fear of school are difficult to treat and may continue to have problems of adjustment.

Depression Depression is signified usually be a generally gloomy lifeless attitude or by a tendency to weep from the slightest cause. This may be accompanied by a change in school performance and a withdrawn and disinterested attitude. When this happens at puberty or adolescence there is a very real danger of suicide and the signs should never, never be ignored. Immediate (meaning on the same day) medical advice must be sought.

Obsessional neurosis Most young children go through a phase of observing rituals such as hopping on every other paving stone, tipping every other railing post and such like. Children with obsessional states appear to have exaggerated ritualistic behaviour sometimes to the exclusion of all else.

After puberty obsessions generally take the form of continual handwashing, sometimes thought to be associated with attempts to clean away some inner moral guilt. Anorexia nervosa is a particularly serious obsession of adolescent and young adult women who become totally immersed in the problem of losing weight because they are figure conscious. They generally start by dieting and eventually reach the stage of either refusing to eat anything or of concealing the fact that they are not eating and if allowed to persist, they will ultimately die.

Hysterics or 'disassociative state' This is when the symptoms of somatic illness are produced as a result of repressed emotional problems or conflicts, thereby disassociating them from the personality. This may extend to periods of loss of vision and hearing and even to paralysis as well as over-ventilation, spasms, odd coughs and a peculiar walking gait. Psychiatric opinion and treatment is needed.

Group 3. Specific Delays and Disorders

These are included in mental health because the physical and emotional aspects are interwoven to an inextricable degree and need to be given equal consideration and be treated together. Children who are late in acquiring skills often demonstrate behaviour disturbance of one kind or another and it is frequently impossible to establish which causes which; is the lateness in acquiring the skill a result of emotional disturbance or vice versa? Parents are often tense and worried about the situation, which in turn affects the child and may further delay development.

Speech Learning in school is not the beginning of learning and a child can only be expected to build on what he already knows. Parents sometimes have the extraordinary idea that school will cure the slow learner and that he will suddenly blossom into a genius. To begin with, a child needs to be able to understand what is going on and to communicate with the teacher and with other children, otherwise he is likely to be left behind the rest of the class and the path to failure and its associated problems is already well under way. Satisfactory speech and language are fundamental to understanding and for this reason the health visitor has a major responsibility to see that the young child is acquiring these skills during the pre-school years.

Satisfactory speech requires the co-ordination of the correct physical movements of the pharynx, soft palate, tongue, lips and muscles of the face, combined with correct breathing. The early feeding habits of the baby and young child are instrumental in developing these physical movements and breathing for satisfactory speech. Having created the conditions for producing sound it is then necessary for the child to have normal hearing and satisfactory brain function to pay attention, listen and gradually comprehend what is being said so that it may be copied and correctly reproduced. Malfunction of any of these mechanisms may cause late, or no development of speech (aphasia) and sometimes a child who has acquired speech may have his ability to express or understand it impaired (dysphasia). Diagnosis requires physical examination and hearing and intelligence testing.

Defective or absent speech should be already under investigation and treated long before a child enters school. However, this is not always the case, and it must be noticed when the child enters school and be brought to the doctor's attention as soon as possible. The commonest faults are as follows:

1. Faulty pronunciation of words, such as lisping or slurring.
2. Using a pattern of speech one would expect of a younger child.
3. Stammering or stuttering.

The speech therapist has an important function to play in helping to diagnose the causes of poor speech development and in planning and carrying out treatment with the child and the parents and also in advising school staff of the correct management. The school doctor and nurse will wish to be in close contact with the speech therapy service.

Language This is the combined use of various methods of interpersonal communication, including speech, gestures and written words. Language difficulties frequently accompany speech problems. However, it should not be assumed that because a child has no speech he is unintelligent and will be unable to communicate. Early silent films, puppets and the theatre of mime demonstrate delightfully the power of human beings to communicate quite complicated concepts without any speech.

The skilful use of language is of a major importance not only as a basis for learning but for establishing relationships and adapting to life generally.

Satisfactory speech combined with good vision and intelligence, comprehension and memory are necessary to language development and any defect in these will hamper progress. Some children have the added advantage of coming from homes where it is part of the life-style for their parents and friends to discuss a variety of topics and abstract ideas using a wide range of vocabulary and methods of expression. These children have usually acquired considerable language ability and are well placed to progress in school although they may not necessarily be particularly intelligent. The health visitor needs to pay attention to this in the pre-school years and see that children have opportunities for language stimulation. Immigrant children may need opportunities to learn English before they go to school if English is not spoken at home. However, the fact that the child does not speak English does not mean that he has not acquired a good concept of the use of language as this will develop according to the range of use he has experienced in his mother-tongue.

Slow learning Speech and language may be fundamental to understanding what is going on in school but they do not necessarily mean that a child is bound to learn and progress. Other difficulties may inhibit him. There may be minor or major physical illnesses or disabilities which prevent him from giving his full attention to the teacher or which necessitate frequent absence from school for treatment. He may be socially inadequate and awkward in his relationships with adults and other children, always saying or doing the wrong thing; this will distress him and lead him to expect to fail in other ways. He may come from a disturbed and unhappy home, which makes him feel miserable and depressed or, perhaps when he is older, ashamed of it.

Possibly, he may be of low intelligence or suffer from neurological effects on the brain caused by birth injury, infection or drugs, which make him over-active and unable to pay attention long enough to learn anything. Sometimes the brain does not seem to be able to interpret the meaning of the written word even though the child may be otherwise intelligent and there is no apparent physical cause. This condition is frequently described as *dyslexia* although there is a great deal of professional controversy about the term and its meaning. In any event such children are generally recognized by their failure to learn to read. They often manage to pick out certain letters or numbers but not a whole word. Written work (see Fig. 17) is generally dotted with spelling mistakes but usually of the kind where letters such as 'b' and 'd' are confused or placed in the wrong order, or a word might either contain extra syllables or be missing them. Often the same word will be correctly and incorrectly spelt or even spelt in several different ways on the same page. Mirror writing is also commonly seen. Such children often copy written work extremely well but when asked to produce it from memory will present a standard of writing and spelling well below what might be expected. This is called dysgraphia. Some children have similar problems with numerical work (dyscalculia) in that they cannot remember multiplication tables, or the sequence of the months of the year.

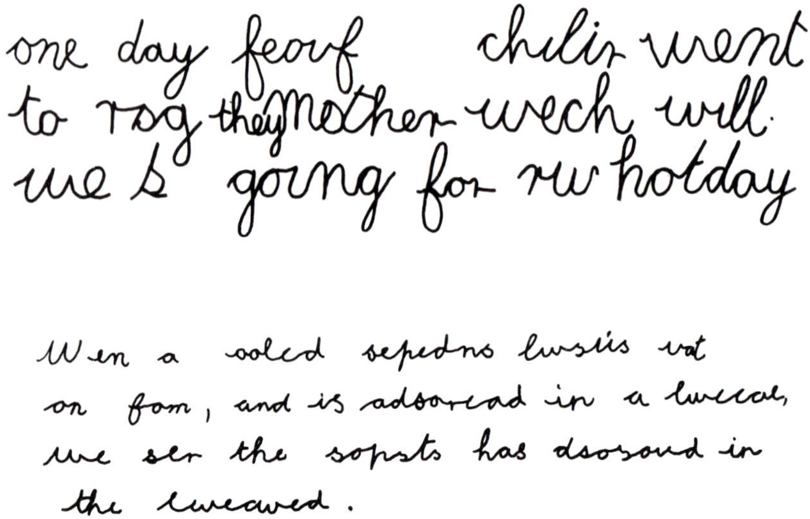

Fig. 17. Two examples of dyslexic handwriting. Top: One day five children went to ask their mother, Where shall we be going for our holiday. Bottom: When a solid substance loses its own form, and is absorbed in a liquid, we say the substance has dissolved in the liquid. (Courtesy of T. R. Miles On Helping the Dyslexic Child *and Methuen & Co. Ltd)*

This kind of work in class is often associated with establishing hand and eye co-ordination or indeed which hand to use. They may be left-handed and right-eyed, or vice versa (cross-laterality), able to use both hands alike (ambidexterity) or they may be left-handed (sinistrality), and often there is a family history of such combinations.

The pre-school health services have a responsibility not only to try to prevent and treat conditions likely to affect future learning but to draw the attention of teachers to children entering school who are likely to be affected by these difficulties. On school entry teachers have a duty to seek the assistance of the school medical team to discover the causes of learning disorders and of planning to alleviate them.

Clumsiness Some children seem to have a great difficulty in tasks such as writing, drawing, ball games and practical work requiring motor skills. When this is accompanied by other symptoms such as hyperactivity, difficulty in paying attention or perception problems, there may be a history of birth trauma or systemic infection which could have resulted in minor brain damage.

Tics Spasms of the body or face are sometimes seen in young children and usually disappear unless associated with other developmental disorders.

Toilet training Problems of enuresis and soiling affect many primary school age children. Loss of sphincter control is a common reaction in all human beings in times of acute stress or anxiety and needs to be recognized as such in a child new to the school who may be shy and frightened. Such a child may also be intimidated by the teacher's attitude to requests to leave the room or indeed may not understand how to make such a request. In older schools the toilet accommodation may be unpleasant, cold or lack the privacy some children need, or there may not be sufficient time allowed for all children to visit the toilet at break periods. Similarly, the toilet arrangements in the home need investigating. Such mundane solutions need to be considered before elaborate investigation is embarked upon.

Enuresis This is quite a common occurrence in children, particularly boys between the ages of 5 and 11 years. It usually happens at night when the child is sleeping and rarely occurs during the day time. Children who continue to wet both during the day and night generally have some physical abnormality. Enuresis in any child over the age of five years needs investigation. It is commoner in children of families in socio-economic class IV and V where there is a family history of bed-wetting. Some doctors believe it can be traced to attempts to potty-train at too early an age or to stressful events around the time when the child would normally be gaining sphincter control (two to three years of age). A thorough examination is needed to exclude physical causes and treatment will depend on the diagnosis. The parents will need reassurance and explanation about the management of the child as well as practical help such as incontinence laundry service. Families living in poor circumstances may need help with extra bedding or the provision of a separate bed for the child. Drug treatment may be prescribed or frequently a pad and buzzer are used. The latter method works on the principle that as soon as the child starts to wet the buzzer sounds and wakes the child who then visits the toilet; eventually the child will wake automatically without the use of the buzzer. Two pads attached to the buzzer by wires are connected as illustrated in Fig. 18. The buzzer is placed in a position which necessitates the child getting out of bed to turn it off. The child then visits the toilet and the bed is re-made. For convenience, draw sheets may be used and pulled through to a dry area and the buzzer is then re-set. This kind of exercise obviously needs reasonably intelligent and co-operative parents as well as a certain amount of privacy for the child, i.e. his own bed. Treatment is usually said to be complete if the child has been dry for three consecutive weeks although the habit may recur and a small percentage of children need a second course of treatment.

Encopresis and faecal soiling This is when small quantities of faeces are dribbled onto the underwear or bed-clothes several times during the day or night, often with a foul embarassing smell. Like enuresis it is more common in boys than girls and should be investigated. The cause may be a physical one resulting in constipation, with incontinent overflow (soiling) or it may be from voluntary

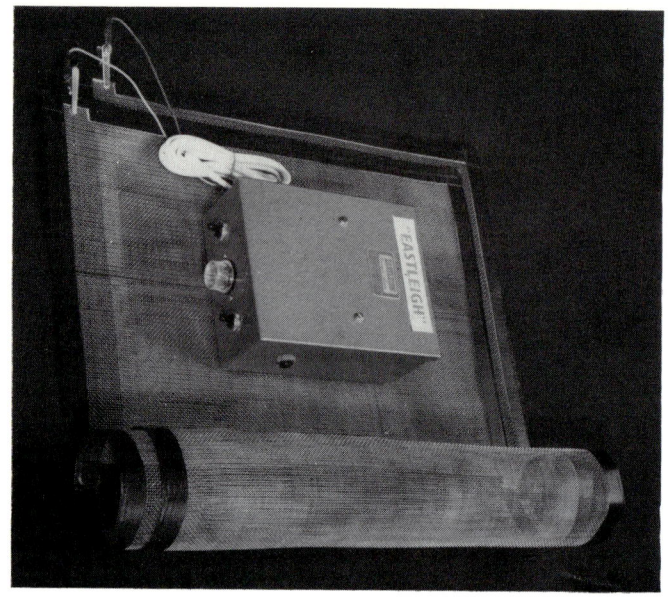

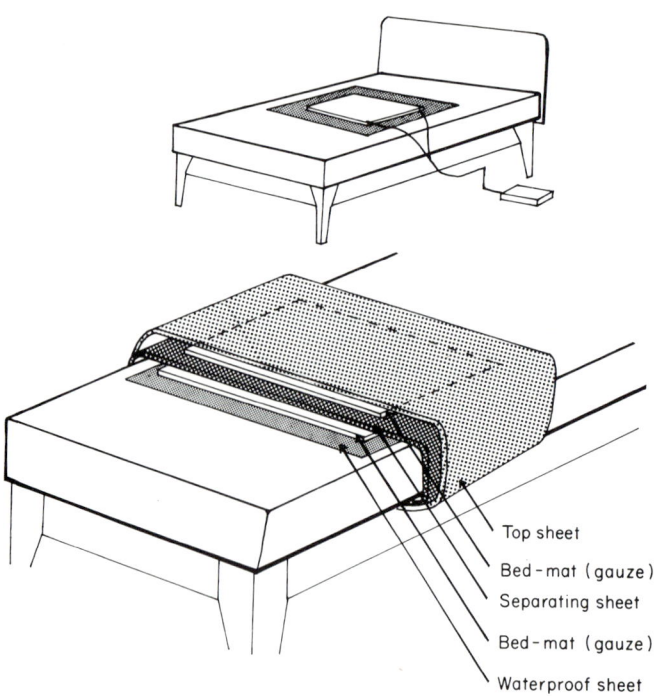

Top sheet

Bed-mat (gauze)

Separating sheet

Bed-mat (gauze)

Waterproof sheet

retention of a normal stool (encopresis) usually as a result of emotional stress. This may be from a temporary disturbance such as the birth of a younger child or a period of marital disharmony. It may also be associated with personality disorder or a distorted relationship between parent and child (usually a very domineering or over-protective parent). This requires investigation and treatment by the child psychiatric team. The prognosis is good and it rarely persists into adolescence.

Eating and sleeping difficulties These are quite common and in young children are usually the result of bad habit formation during the pre-school years. Sometimes they are attention-seeking ploys known to attract immediate reaction. Providing there is nothing physically the matter with a child, exercise and reasonable sleeping conditions ought to promote sleep. Eating habits should improve if all snacks between meals are stopped and if food not eaten within the meal-time is thrown away. Older children under emotional stress may over-eat to compensate or under-eat in an effort to slim.

Group 4. Psychosis

This is characterized by behaviour which bears no relation to normality or reality. This is most likely to occur during a high fever caused by severe systemic infection, such as meningitis, and is unlikely to be of long-term significance. Childhood autism, although comparatively rare, is long-term and usually starts before the age of two years. These children seem to live in a world of their own and generally resent physical and emotional contact. They spend their time performing very exaggerated rituals such as twisting round and round, banging the head and rocking. Because it is almost impossible to make contact with them, they usually fail to learn even basic speech and language although their IQ may be normal or even high and they are not usually deaf. Many of them are fond of music and this may be one way of reaching them in endeavouring to make contact and to teach them. About half of them end up in hospitals for the mentally handicapped. Adolescents may develop psychosis which usually takes the form of schizophrenia or severe depression.

SCHOOL RESPONSIBILITIES

The school's function in relation to mental health is three-fold:

1. To provide an emotionally secure, stable and supportive community.
2. Provision of personnel sufficiently skilled to diagnose and devise suitable treatment and education (child psychiatric team).

Fig. 18. Pad and buzzer; the alarm is connected to opposite corners of the bed-mats. (Courtesy of N. H. Eastwood & Sons Ltd, 70 Nursery Road, Southgate London N.14)

3. To provide education for the prevention of mental breakdown in future generations.

School Size and Organization

The provision of an emotionally stable and supportive community for each individual child presents something of a problem, particularly in very large schools. This is further compounded where the children come from unstable changing communities and the teaching staff are transient. Most of us will remember the feeling of bewilderment and uncertainty during the first days in a new school and how gradually one acquired a group of friends and particular rapport with certain teachers. Some of us have memories of school as a place where life-long friends were made, happy, eager days which influenced our thoughts and actions and provided us with the basis of many of the pleasures we enjoy today. Some remember it as a place where weaknesses were highlighted and pounced upon by other children who teased and taunted relentlessly, classes were boring and each day was purgatory. Most of us probably have memories reflecting both sides of the picture.

The school has a responsibility to provide a structure in which children can make friends and develop a good rapport with caring adults. There are a variety of ways of trying to provide this. Generally, some of the teachers are given special responsibility for the children's 'pastoral' care, i.e. seeking out, guiding and counselling the child in difficulties, together with making contact with supportive agencies as necessary (health team and social services). In primary schools this is usually the class teacher. Secondary schools, particularly large comprehensive schools of some 2000 children, may have various systems, the most common one being the house system in which children from all age groups will belong to an individual house unit headed by a house master to whom a number of house tutors will be responsible. Each house tutor will have charge and continue to have responsibilities for a group of children of the same age (horizontal grouping) or of varying ages (vertical grouping) throughout their school lives.

The teaching profession is divided in its attitude to pastoral care, some believing that this vocational aspect should be combined with subject work, as problems need to be dealt with as they arise, and some feeling that counselling is specialist work requiring at least a one-year special course. Others are of the opinion that counselling is not necessarily a teacher's function and so some education authorities appoint nurses full-time in schools believing them, particularly those with families and of a motherly nature, to be well-suited to this work. They may well be right and it is an aspect of nursing as yet untested and about which we know virtually nothing and have certainly not attempted to prepare nurses for. Recognition of the possibilities has, however, been given in the Court Report[1] which suggests that where possible this type of nurse should be appointed full-time in secondary schools.

Whatever the system, the school health team need to be in constant contact with those responsible for this aspect of the child's care. To facilitate communication some schools have set up pastoral care teams or committees which meet regularly and discuss any children who may be presenting problems. Personnel such as house masters, probation officers, education welfare officers and social workers, psychologists and psychiatrists, school doctors and nurses, and perhaps members of the board of governors, might belong to such groups. Particularly attention needs to be paid to children known to be under stress such as:

1. Family crisis; divorce, illness or death.
2. Parent with psychiatric illness or severe emotional problems.
   These first two groups are also situations when children are most likely to be physically battered as their parents are under stress.
3. Entry to new school or class, particularly a child who does not proceed with his classmates. Also the child of an immigrant family newly arrived in this country.
4. Following a long period of illness of absence from school.
5. Puberty and the related upheavals of sexual and social adjustment.
6. Pending academic examinations.

Primary–Secondary Transfer

Communication between primary and secondary schools is important and to facilitate this some authorities are arranging for certain groups of primary schools to 'feed' the local secondary school, though this should not inhibit the free choice of parents. Where this system functions, nurse staffing might be adjusted to a similar pattern to maintain continuity.

Counselling

In practice children generally select their own counsellors and, therefore, there should be suitable people sufficiently well-known and available to whom they can take their worries. This may well be an appointed counsellor, a teacher, the school nurse or doctor, the social worker or educational welfare officer, provided the right kind of people occupy these posts. However, it may just as easily be the school helper, first-aider, or caretaker. Equally, some children avoid adults and need to be sought out and a relationship actively established. Examples have been seen over the last few years of children who have committed suicide as a result of being persistently bullied while no adult in the school or home appeared to be aware of the degree of stress suffered by them. House tutors or year-masters have a special duty to make themselves aware of such happenings. Additionally, part of the youth service responsibility includes frequenting places where adolescents meet in order to make contact with them. In any event, everyone in school needs to be sufficiently aware of children's needs to know when to seek advice and to whom to refer the child.

Diagnosis and Treatment

The services of an educational psychologist should be available to children with learning difficulties at an early date. He will want the opinion of the school doctor to exclude medical causes and together with the social worker and education welfare officer he is likely to deal with a number of children. Some children, however, need the attention of the complete child psychiatric team which includes the child psychiatrist, the educational psychologist, the psychiatric social worker and the child psychotherapist. They will endeavour to work together with the parents and the child to devise a suitable programme of treatment and education.

Various individual or combined measures may be taken depending on the over-riding problem (it is seldom that one is found in isolation), the circumstances of the child and the family and the range and choice of provision available. Children with speech and language problems need the help of a qualified speech therapist who may visit the school or the child and his parents may have to attend the speech therapy clinic. The teacher of the deaf and partially hearing will, of course, be involved if there is a hearing problem.

Remedial teaching Slow learners may attend special remedial teaching classes, generally conducted in the school by a remedial teacher. Where this is insufficient and the child is generally a 'slow learner' arrangements may have to be made for him to attend a school for educationally subnormal children, either for a period of time or for the rest of his school life depending on his progress.

Maladjusted Severely disturbed children may need to attend a school for maladjusted children. This may be daily or, if it is thought that the child would benefit from a period away from home, residential schools may be considered or hostel accommodation might be arranged by the social services department. This kind of provision has considerable implications for families and the attachment of a child to his family may be weakened by long absences from home. Therefore, every effort is needed to see that the family is not broken up and that work proceeds either in the child's absence or with the family group in the residential home, to sufficiently improve the management of the situation for the child to return home as soon as possible.

A few children need hospital care, preferably in a day unit if it is available. A proportion of children will require in-patient treatment. Staff working with disturbed children need considerable skill in understanding the causes of the child's behaviour and in reacting appropriately. Anger and despair may be expressed by violent kicking and biting and this may alternate with clinging sobbing spells. This usually requires firm calm restraining while talking to the child and followed by cuddling. Continuity of relationships with certain members of staff is encouraged. Methods of behaviour therapy are used with the guidance of the child psychiatrist. Good behaviour is rewarded and aggression is as far as possible diverted into physical activities, practical work, painting and drama. This work is hard and arduous and the results are not always rewarding. Some children are so unmanageable that they can no longer be contained in school and alternative care has to be found for them.

To Educate for Future Prevention

While not all problems are preventable, a large proportion would be avoided if parents had a better knowledge of children's needs and this was applied to their early care. Equally, the early use of health services for family planning, abortion, genetic counselling, antenatal and maternity care would reduce both the stress of unwanted children and the risk of traumas and birth injuries so often affecting the physical and mental development of the child. The education service, therefore, has a responsibility to see that children in school are equally well prepared for the important job of being parents as they are for earning a living. As outlined in Chapter 11 the health service must assist them in their efforts and demonstrate the value of their own services.

REFERENCES

1. Court Report (1976) *Fit for the Future—Report of the Committee on Child Health Services*. London: HMSO, Cmnd 6684.

FURTHER READING

Barker, P. (1976) *Basic Child Psychiatry*, 2nd ed. St Albans: Crosby Lockwood Staples.
Brierley, J. (1976) *The Growing Brain*. Windsor, Berkshire: N.F.E.R. Publ. Co.
Emotional Problems in Childhood and Adolescence (1973) Selection of articles published in the *Br. med. J*.
DHSS *The Family in Society—Dimensions of Parenthood* (1974) London: HMSO.
Laslett, R. ed. (1970) *Day Schools for Maladjusted Children*. An account by a group of head teachers in the Greater London Area. London: Association of Workers for Maladjusted Children.
Miles, T. R. (1974) *The Dyslexic Child*. London: Methuen.
Gale, B. (1975) *Pastoral Care—Report of the Working Party on Pastoral Care Arrangements in Secondary Schools*. Winchester: Hampshire Education Authority.
Pinkerton, P. (November 1975—July 1976) Series on Child Psychiatry. *Nursing Mirror*.
Tizard Report (1972) *Children with Specific Reading Difficulties—Report of the Advisory Committee on Handicapped Children*. London: DES, HMSO.
Varma, V. P. (1973) *Stresses in Children*. London: U. L. P. Particularly related to children in school.

CHILDREN'S BOOKS

Non-fiction
Showers, P. (1976) *Sleep is for Everyone*. London: Black. 5+ years.

Fiction

Ashley, B. (1974) *Trouble with Donovan Croft*. Oxford: Oxford University Press. Donovan has to be fostered while his mother returns to the West Indies. He is so unhappy he refuses to speak and is seen by the educational psychologist in school. 10+ years.

Gydal, M. & Danielsson, T. (1976) *When Olly's Grandad Died*. Sevenoaks: Hodder & Stoughton. Describes Olly's relationship with grand-dad and what happens when he dies. 6+ years.

Gydal, M. & Danielsson, T. (1976) *When Gemma's Parents Got Divorced*. Sevenoaks: Hodder & Stoughton. Gemma's parents keep quarrelling, they separate and new families are formed. 6+ years.

Mary, M. (1974) *Stepmother*. The 'wicked stepmother' turns out to be not so bad after all. 4+ years.

Sen, Felicity (1975) *My Family*. London: Bodley Head. How father and two children cope alone. 3+ years.

Spence, E. (1976) *October Child*. Oxford: Oxford University Press. The long-awaited new baby is autistic and the effect on the family is disastrous. 11+ years.

USEFUL ADDRESSES AND INFORMATION

Mind (National Association for Mental Health)
22 Harley Street
London W1.
Tel: 01 637 0741.

Information, advice, seminars on all aspects of mental health.

The National Association for the Gifted Child
1 South Audley Street
London W1.
Tel: 01 499 1188.

Provides information and advice.

The National Youth Bureau
17–23 Albion Street
Leicester LE1 6GD.
Tel: 0533 (Leicester) 53 8811.

Offers free enquiry service on all aspects of youth, together with loan of teaching materials to assist in training professionals. Publishes a bi-monthly journal *Youth in Society*.

Discussion Topics

1. A child's behaviour pattern has suddenly totally changed. Consider any reasons which might have caused this to happen and the support which might be given in each case.

2. A fourteen-year-old is absent from school. Later it is established that he was admitted to hospital following attempted suicide by taking an overdose of drugs. Discuss the various possible reasons for this, the system of prevention in the school and the various follow-up possibilities which might be considered.

3. A teacher reports a child to be a 'slow learner'. What role will the school nurse play in his assessment?

4. A teenager is frequently absent from school. Consider the possible causes and solutions.

5. Consider the problem of the enuretic child in (a) a day school, (b) residential school, (c) going on the school journey. In what ways could the school nurse be of most assistance?

6. 'Prevention is better than cure'. What preventive measures in relation to mental health might the school nurse be actively associated with in school?

8
The Handicapped Child

According to Chambers English Dictionary, 'to handicap' means 'to impose special disadvantages or impediments'. Many children are in just such a position for various reasons and to varying degrees. Indeed it has been said that one in seven of all school children has a condition of sufficient severity to affect their education prospects.

Advances in medicine have meant that more children with physical defects or brain damage survive through school age into adulthood. Other children have been born into such socially disadvantaged circumstances that they never receive the intellectual stimulation, or perhaps the emotional security, required for their personality and intellect to grow and develop. Like young plants in adverse conditions they survive in a stunted fashion.

The child with one handicap is likely to have others, and even a child of good intelligence must face the consequent delays and obstructions imposed on living and normal development. Additionally, the child has to adjust to the world and to the sort of problems he or she can expect as an adult which places heavy demands on mental health, and behaviour disturbances or mal-adjustment may well arise. It is, therefore, important that no time is lost in detecting handicap or delay at the earliest possible age so that suitable medical and educational treatment may be embarked upon. The importance of parents' role in encouraging and supporting the child must be recognized and advice and instruction be made available to them so that they are adequately equipped to help their child in the best possible way.

Education is concerned with developing natural talents so that life may be as satisfying as possible. Therefore, for handicapped children, special facilities and teaching skills are needed either to help them overcome or to cope with their particular disability and live as satisfactory a life as possible. Prevention and early detection of handicap is a prime function of the child health service as a whole and the school health service team have an important part to play with their education colleagues in assessing and planning the special educational needs of the handicapped child.

Handicap register In order to assist in the administration of the services for handicapped children and to ensure continuous surveillance, a register of handicapped children is maintained by the area specialist in child health. Children are placed on that register by a senior child health doctor as soon as handicap is established.

Prevention

The hazards and mistakes of one generation need not necessarily be repeated in the next and this ought to be foremost in our minds, particularly in schools, because it is here that many of the attitudes and patterns for adult life will be formed. Medical advances have not only succeeded in keeping more handicapped children alive but also in discovering the causes of many handicapping conditions. There is increasing interest in the prevention of handicapping conditions and it is of the utmost importance that children who are the next generation of parents understand the advantages of preventive measures such as genetic counselling, family planning advice and immunization and vaccination. Indeed, rubella vaccination is a major advance in the prevention of handicapping conditions, but as yet the uptake is disappointingly low. Early use of maternity and child health services are important, particularly during the antenatal period. For example, for parents with a family history of chromosomal abnormalities, an obstetric history of spina bifida, or if the mother is over the age of 30 years and therefore at greater risk of producing a child with Down's Syndrome, a test of the amniotic fluid (amniocentesis) may be suggested to the mother and if evidence of handicap is found, abortion may be offered.

Comprehensive Assessment

Congenital defect or handicap may either be obvious at birth and be diagnosed by the paediatrician following delivery or it may become apparent at a later date through the health visitors and child health doctors' pre-school developmental screening. It is then necessary for the child to have a full diagnostic assessment, and a suitable programme of treatment and education should begin. The district general hospital is usually the most likely place for a range of diagnostic equipment and specialists to be found and, therefore, this kind of assessment is usually based there, particularly for the pre-school child. The assessment team will include a senior or consultant paediatrician, a specialist social worker, a principal clinical or educational psychologist, a health visitor or nursing officer with special expertise in handicap and a teacher. Other professionals such as the audiologist, speech therapist and physiotherapist will be included as appropriate. They will also need the assistance of pertinent observations from parents and staff closely associated with the child. The questions the team have to ask and answer are what exactly are this child's difficulties and what are the causes? How are we to treat him medically and how are we to combine this with the optimum opportunities to learn so that he may be equipped in every possible way to cope with adult life?

Special Education

The local education authority has a duty to provide education for all children in the area irrespective of their circumstances. Legally they are required to provide education for a handicapped child from the age of two years but many forward-thinking education authorities are planning and providing educational input before that. For instance, a teacher of the deaf will start work with a partially-hearing child's parents when the child is six to nine months. Recommendations for special education were largely the doctors' responsibility until 1975 when the responsibility for the final decision was placed with the educational psychologist although the decision is based on the consensus of the comprehensive assessment team. Documentation for the purpose was also introduced in 1975. These are Special Education Forms SE1–SE6 which are completed by various members of the team although to date their use does not seem to be very successful and consequently it is being reconsidered.

In recent years there has been considerable controversy as to where and how special facilities should be provided, the most recent legislation being the 1976 Education Act, Section 10. This amends the 1944 Education Act in relation to pupils requiring special educational treatment in that provision for this must now be made in county or voluntary schools other than where it is (a) 'impracticable or incompatible with the provision of efficient instruction in the schools, or (b) would involve unreasonable public expenditure when arrangements may be made for children to attend special schools'.

In the main, these special schools have evolved since 1945 when the Department of Education and Science drew up the following list of categories:

> Blind.
> Partially-sighted.
> Deaf.
> Partially-hearing.
> Educationally subnormal (slow learners ESN).
> Epileptic.
> Maladjusted.
> Physically handicapped.
> Speech defect.
> Delicate (chest and heart complaints).

These are still in use although the patterns of disease have changed considerably. There are now far fewer children with untreatable chest and heart complaints such as tuberculosis, while the majority of epileptic children can be sufficiently controlled to attend ordinary school. Additionally, since 1971 education authorities have been required to provide education for severely mentally handicapped children now known as severely subnormal (SSN) who until then were the responsibility of the DHSS and cared for by the health service, usually in hospital.

The whole situation is obviously very much in need of review and as mentioned in Chapter 1, a government enquiry under the chairmanship of Mrs Mary Warnock is still, at the time of writing, considering the whole question of special education. The National Children's Bureau suggested in their report *Living with Handicap, 1970* a new list of categories more appropriate to present-day circumstances which will no doubt be considered by the Warnock Committee. They are as follows:

> Visual handicap.
> Hearing impairment.
> Physical handicap.
> Speech and language disorder.
> Specific learning disorder.
> Intellectual handicap.
> Emotional handicap.
> Severe personality disorder.
> Severe environmental handicap.
> Severe multi-handicap.

Not all children with a similar handicap will respond to the same circumstances. Some will need the intellectual competition of ordinary school and be able to adapt happily and socialize with normal children; others are totally unable to cope with the stress of keeping up in normal school and may need the protection and extra facilities of a special school as well as the social support of children with similar difficulties. Some children need a mixture of both or a year or two of special school until they are sufficiently confident to return to normal school. The very severely physically or mentally handicapped may require residential facilities or even long-term hospital care. Special medical and educational facilities may at present be provided in the following circumstances:

1. Ordinary school (head-teacher will decide if suitable education can be provided and the advice of the doctor and nurse will be needed as to the feasibility of providing suitable medical and nursing support).
2. Ordinary school with resource room.
3. Special classes in ordinary school.
4. Special units attached to ordinary school.

5. Full or part-time attendance at special day school.
6. Residential school.
7. Day school with hostel or foster care arrangements provided by the social services.
8. Hospital with schooling facilities attached.
9. Home tuition.

Handicapped children require more individual attention depending on the severity of the handicap and consequently the pupil-teacher ratio is much smaller than that of ordinary school. Peripatetic teachers who specialize in methods suitable for particular handicaps are usually employed to visit and provide advice and help to teachers and pupils in ordinary schools or special schools with multi-handicapped children. Some education authorities are unable to provide such a wide and expensive range of services for comparatively few children; consequently, they can pay for the child to attend a suitable school in another authority or an independent school funded privately or by a voluntary organization.

The Role of the School Nurse

This will differ considerably according to the type of school she is employed in and the range of handicap she encounters. Children who are physically handicapped may need practical nursing care frequently to the extent of accompanying the children on school journeys and holidays (see Fig. 19). Children who are mildly mentally handicapped and who represent some 50% of the educationally subnormal group show a higher incidence of behaviour disorders and minor physical disabilities, for which a nursing background in child psychiatry would be particularly valuable. Those who are severely mentally handicapped are often multi-handicapped with any number of disabilities such as cerebral palsy, incontinence, immobility, epilepsy and behaviour disturbances requiring a wide range of expertise in nursing. Multi-handicapped children have such a variety of special needs that a nurse caring for such children needs to be prepared to acquire a working knowledge of the skills of other professionals such as the physiotherapist, speech therapist and occupational therapist, while at the same time teaching them some of her own expertise. Nurses may need to take part in programmes devised by teachers and therapists and teachers need to know how to cope with emergencies such as epileptic seizures and asthmatic attacks.

The following is a broad outline of nursing responsibilities:

1. Assessing whether suitable nursing care and support can be provided.
2. Teaching care staff and providing information to teachers and support and advice to parents.
3. Liaising with colleagues so that suitable support may be continued during school closure and holiday periods.

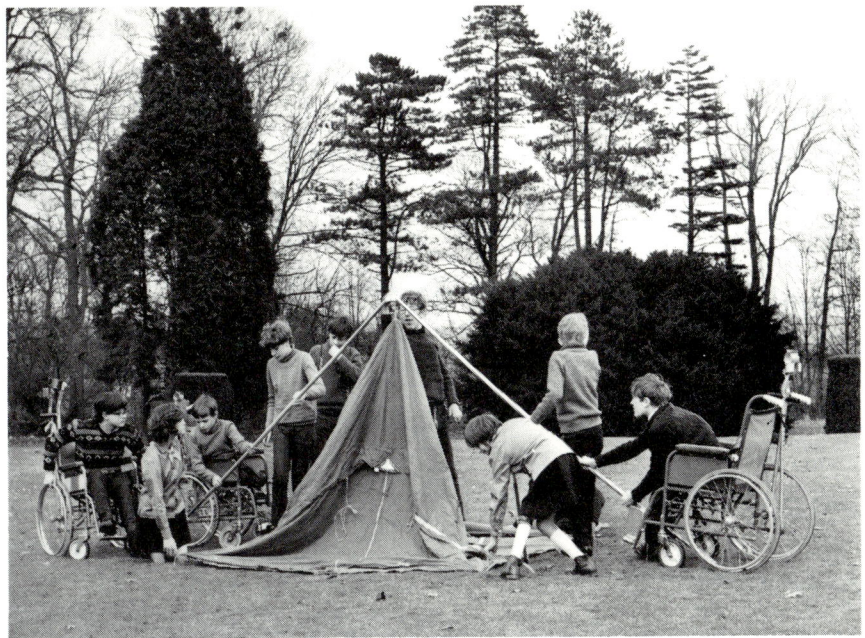

Fig. 19. Physically handicapped children learning to pitch a tent. They are also encouraged to take part in sports such as sailing, riding, archery and games. (Central Office of Information)

4. Preparation and follow-up for medical examinations.
5. Nursing treatments and points of attention.

Assessing whether suitable nursing care and support can be provided This is particularly important when placement in ordinary school is being considered. A physically handicapped child may need nursing attention regularly in school or on occasions. For example, a child with a stoma may be able to manage but there will be occasions when nursing attention is needed. Suitable accommodation should be available so that nursing care can be administered in privacy and the child can rest and be quiet if necessary. It may not be possible for a visiting school nurse, responsible for several primary schools, to be available daily to carry out treatment for one particular child. Consequently, regular nursing may be carried out by the home nursing service depending on the school nurse's commitments. Alternatively, a school helper or teacher may be available and willing to administer care following instruction. The feasibility of the parent visiting the school to undertake treatment might also be discussed. These various possibilities ought to be considered before any child who may require nursing is placed in a school with only a visiting nurse service.

The structure of the school is also important. A child in a wheelchair must be able to move freely round the school and use the toilets. Modern school buildings are now designed with this in mind but in most older buildings this would be impossible without considerable structural alterations. Under certain circumstances the local education authority may be prepared to fit ramps, widen doors and supply suitable furniture. The child may also need assistance in moving round the school, using the toilet, at meal-times and during physical education and recreation.

Residential and special day schools for physically handicapped children usually have full-time nursing and care staff and the school buildings and time-tables are planned to cope with ambulatory and nursing needs.

Teaching care staff and providing information to teachers and support and advice to parents Lay staff are usually employed to help the children in class and with moving around the school and using the toilet. In residential schools they assist the children in washing and dressing in the morning and in preparations for bed at night-time. They should aim to provide in the school all the daily care and mothering that the parent gives in the home. They need guidance in the handling and management required by individual children; for example, how to lift correctly for the benefit and protection of themselves and the child. They also need to know the consequences of infections for certain children and how to give first-aid generally and in circumstances likely to occur, such as asthmatic attacks. Like parents and nurses, they may be inclined to do too much for the child rather than encourage and help him to learn to care for himself.

Teachers, particularly in ordinary schools, may be very fearful of accepting a handicapped child in their class. They may have no idea of the meaning of medical terms and the implications for the child, the class, or the teaching programme, and consequently, explanations and advice as to what to expect are usually welcomed. Many of the voluntary organizations interested in particular disabilities publish excellent leaflets and booklets specially designed for teachers and parents and the school nurse ought to see that they are available and explained by the doctor or nurse.

Parents will come to the school and opportunities should be sought to show them how to maintain care during evenings, weekends and holidays. The practicabilities of coping are often not explained to them or they are not given opportunities to practise under supervision which many parents would welcome. This will, all too frequently, result in the child being mismanaged and bored at home, often returning to school having deteriorated considerably after a long holiday. This usually means that neither the parents nor the child have particularly enjoyed the experience, which does not help their future relationships.

Liaising with colleagues Parents are not always capable of coping and may need professional continuous support while the child is at home. Neglect during this time can undo much of the work achieved in the school. A bright but physically handicapped child has been known to lose one year's schooling through neglect of pressure areas over a weekend.

The nurse who is attending a child at home needs some background knowledge of what has gone on in school, what the child is capable of performing for himself and what sort of care the school nurse has had to provide. It is obviously more satisfactory for nurses to have direct dialogue with each other though this may be difficult if the child attends school in one area and lives in another. Requests for holiday nursing are usually referred direct to the family practitioner or to the area health authority. However, there is no reason why a school nurse cannot include a letter to her nursing colleague. Alternatively, the area nurse (child health) may be contacted to deal with any queries or to act as a referral point. The *Health Services Year Book* contains the names and addresses of every area nurse (child health) throughout the country and a current copy is usually available in the local administration office.

Preparation and follow-up for medical examinations Handicapped children usually require more frequent medical examination, either by the school doctor or specialist consultant who may visit the school; the usual preparation of records, test results or screenings as required should be made. Follow-up and hospital appointments may need to be arranged either by the nurse, education welfare officer or social worker, as appropriate.

Nursing treatments and points of attention A variety of nursing treatments may need to be carried out by the nurse, the child or the parent. Consequently, it is a nursing responsibility to see that a child can manage such procedures as injections (see Fig. 20), care of a stoma, urine and bowel functions, as soon as possible. The nurse needs to be adept at assessing what the child can be expected to achieve and do for himself, and what is totally beyond him. While caring for one's body is an important part of learning to be independent, insistence may cause distress and discourage the child. A child who is slow in learning in class is likely to be slow in learning to do other things; consequently, the teacher's advice and observations are helpful. Often the nurse and teacher can beneficially work together. The reasons for injections, their effects and administration can become an absorbing part of biology, mathematics or chemistry lessons. They are all the more applicable because the children will be interested and more likely to co-operate with the nurse's instructions. The nurse may be able to supply additional visual aids in the way of used X-rays from the local hospital, testing sticks and papers for urine, or items of nursing equipment, all of which can be used by the teacher in class. An additional advantage of such an approach is that much of the child's anxiety may be relieved by open discussion and many of the unasked questions will be answered automatically during the lesson.

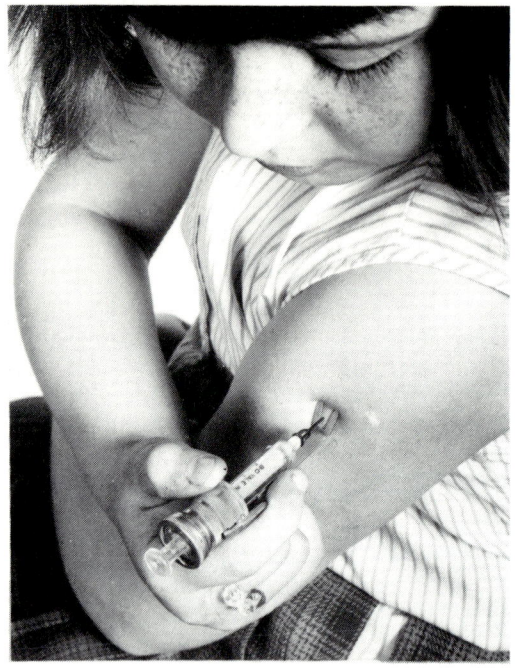

Fig. 20. A diabetic child giving her own injection and so learning to be independent.

Areas for nursing attention can be listed under the following topics.

1. *Supervision of drugs* Teachers vary in their attitudes to dispensing drugs to children in school. Some regard it as part of their overall pastoral care and others feel it is outside their range of duties. Teachers' professional organizations are very opposed to their members accepting responsibility as they recognize the vulnerable position of teachers dispensing drugs given to them in envelopes or wrapped in paper handkerchiefs. Where possible doctors should prescribe treatment which can be administered outside school hours by the parents. The policy for medication in acute circumstances such as an infected wound is very different from chronic conditions such as epilepsy or diabetes where a child needs medicine at specific times to control the condition. Suitable arrangements need to be discussed and made before the child is accepted at an ordinary school. Where there is a permanent nurse she should see that there is written permission from the parents to dispense the drugs. Children should have their own drugs labelled and kept in the containers issued to them by the pharmacy. Pharmacists are not allowed to issue one prescription in two separate containers; therefore, in order that a supply may be kept in school and in the home, two prescriptions may be needed. To avoid

duplication, a record should be kept of all drugs as soon as they are dispensed. They should be kept in a securely locked cupboard and as they are the property of the child they should be given to the parents when the child leaves the school. The parents should be advised to return them to the pharmacy for correct disposal if they are no longer required. Under no circumstances should nurses issue drugs from stock bottles or dispense supplies to parents or teachers in spare containers. Teachers need to be warned when drugs or drug dosage has been changed so that they can report any effects such as drowsiness in class, giddiness, or somatic symptoms.

2. *Eyes and ears* Defects of sight and hearing may occur as a single handicap, or they frequently accompany others. Whatever the circumstances they should not be neglected, and it is depressing to find multi-handicapped children not using glasses or hearing aids which might add something, however small, to their already restricted learning dimensions. Nurses must pay special attention to see that appliances are used, fitting and functioning and that there are no unnecessary delays in repair or replacement (see Chapters 5 and 6). Infections and discharges need attention and treatment, and regular vision screening should be carried out.

3. *Skin* The care of the skin is extremely important, particularly if a child is using calipers, a prosthesis or a wheelchair. Children grow quickly and appliances may become too small and start chaffing and rubbing, causing irritation and breakdown of the skin. Consequently, immobile children need to have pressure areas regularly inspected and treated. The body temperature control may be affected if limbs are missing and sweating may cause irritation and rashes; therefore, attention needs to be given to the type of clothing materials worn. Generally, natural fibres such as cotton and wool are more absorbent and less likely to cause irritation or discomfort.

4. *Kidney and bladder functions* Incontinence of urine is a constant threat to healthy skin and suitable steps to protect it need to be taken. A child who is likely to develop bladder control with careful training is unlikely to benefit from indwelling catheters although if one is used a suitable design which does not need constant renewal with the inevitable risks of infection should be chosen. Boys, of course, are easier to manage by attaching polyethene appliances to the penis. One-way nappies or pads allowing urine to pass through but keeping the surface of the skin dry may be helpful and there are a wide selection of waterproof pants and incontinence pads which may be used. These are ordered through area health authority supplies.

Some children may have stomas to be cared for and a practical guide suitable for nurses or parents entitled *The Care of an Ileal Conduit and Urinary Appliances* is published by the Spina Bifida Association. This publication also includes excellent advice on problems such as swimming, travelling and other complications which may arise. Fluid intake and output may need to be measured and observed for colour and smell as infections (even among normal girls) are quite common.

5. *Bowels* Immobile children suffer considerably from constipation; consequently, diet and motions need attention. High colonic constipation may provoke symptoms of nausea, vomiting and general malaise and while washouts, enemas and suppositories may need to be resorted to, it is preferable to adjust the diet correctly. Care staff ought to be alerted to the children likely to have problems so that they can pay special attention to the frequency of motions and sometimes regular use of the toilet can help to ease the difficulty. School journeys and outings may be somewhat of an ordeal for children with poor sphincter control and this can be avoided if the trouble is anticipated and suitable precautions taken to cope with any incontinence.

6. *Diet and feeding* Children will become obese if they are regularly eating large meals and taking little exercise. Bored children may eat to fill in the time though this ought not to be the case in school at least. Often the fault lies with parents who overfeed their children to compensate for other things they feel they are missing. These parents require advice and guidance. Special schools usually have their own kitchens and are used to providing special diets, so it is easy to produce an alternative meal at short notice for the child with diarrhoea or constipation. Ordinary schools where meals are delivered from a central kitchen are another matter and school helpers need to know what arrangements they can make in emergencies. Local education authorities may have dieticians involved in planning the school meal service; however, advice from the dietician attached to the hospital where a child has been treated is probably best. Severely handicapped children, especially those with cerebral palsy, demonstrating spastic or athetoid movements, have particular problems in learning to control feeding implements. Excessive tongue thrust and salivation makes it difficult to retain the food in the mouth and reduces its consistency to a wet soggy mess, unless suitable textures of food are chosen. Where feeding is a particular problem, all the staff should be involved because learning the correct basic biting and chewing movements is essential for the development of intelligible speech as well as teeth, gums and jaws. Early dental care and treatment is also essential. This is often neglected and some handicapped children suffer severe decay and facial deformity through absence of suitable professional attention. The physiotherapist or occupational therapist and speech therapist will advise and demonstrate the feeding techniques to be used. Whatever the circumstances, meals should be a pleasurable event and children who are slow or find it difficult need to be given encouragement and time.

7. *Control of infection* For some children contact with infectious diseases may be fatal. Children having chemotherapy for the treatment of cancers such as leukaemia, will have practically no resistance to infection. Therefore, contact with outbreaks of measles and other diseases should be avoided. Any such

contact should be notified immediately to the doctor and the consultant treating the child.

Children having physiotherapy, as for example with cystic fibrosis, may easily develop pneumonia or bronchitis if therapy ceases for some reason. It is therefore important that another therapist is found or alternative arrangements made.

8. *Lifting* Poor lifting techniques may cause damage or fractures to very deformed spastic children or those with brittle or structurally weak bones, for example in cases of osteoporosis. Sometimes fractures may remain undetected if the child feels no pain. The physiotherapist is generally the best person to advise on techniques to be adopted with individual children.

9. *Appliances* Alternatives have to be found for missing skills, and shoes, supports, special corsets and calipers need to be specially fitted to the needs of individual children. Specialist appliance fitters undertake this in consultation with the physiotherapist and the consultant. Firms do differ in what they will make for individual children as, for example, cosmetic calipers which are available but are not supplied by all appliance manufacturers. Wheelchairs are equally important, and it is not always sufficient to order a standard model suitable for a child as this may not be adequate for the disability; it may not be comfortable to use or convenient to handle. Nurses or care staff in constant contact with children are most likely to notice faults or hear complaints from the children about appliances or wheelchairs, and should see that these are immediately brought to the attention of the doctor or physiotherapist in touch with the fitter at the DHSS appliance centre.

10. *Aids and clothing* To be as independent as possible is an important aim for every handicapped child and there are now a large variety of aids available, ranging from specially designed baths, beds and telephones to individual small items such as tooth-brushes and feeding utensils. Indeed, the scope is enormous. Clothing too may be designed to be up-to-date, fashionable and yet adapted to enable ease in dressing and undressing (Fig. 21 top), while also meeting individual requirements, as shown in Fig. 21 bottom. Other examples include detachable bib fronts for children constantly salivating or dribbling food, additional padding to avoid chaffing from harnesses, or extra gussets to disguise skeletal malformation. The Disabled Living Foundation have a special interest and expertise in all aspects of aids and clothing and will provide verbal and written information, and often a speaker on request.

11. *Emergencies* Handicapped children tend to be more accident-prone and suitable first-aid arrangements should be made not only for general accidents but for specific emergencies likely to arise with certain diseases. All the staff should know how to act in a crisis and there should be a clear policy on calling medical assistance and of knowing where the child is to be sent if immediate admission to hospital is required. For example, a child with a blocked Spitz

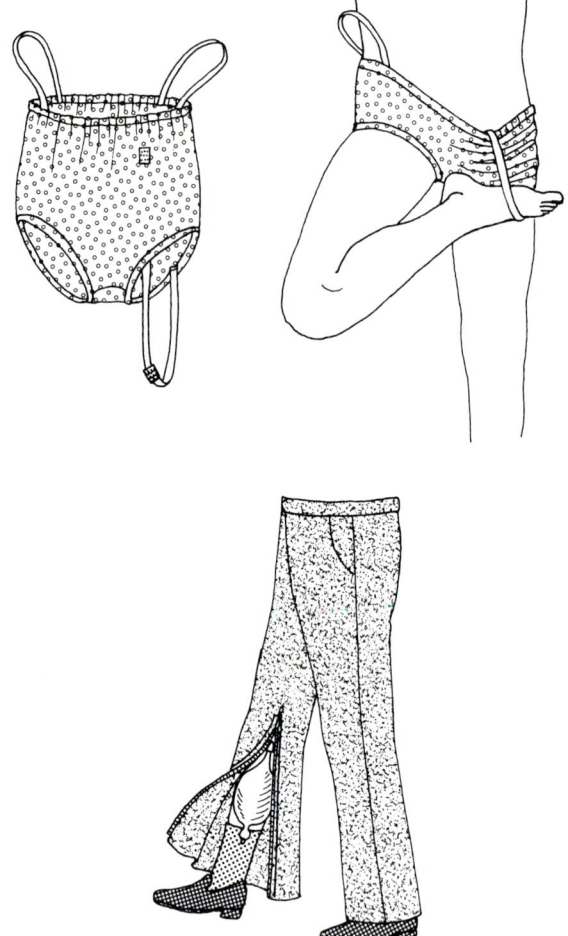

Fig. 21. Top: *A loop tape enables pants to be pulled down with toes, thereby encouraging independence;* Bottom: *a zip inserted in a trouser leg enables urine bag strapped to the leg to be emptied easily.* (*Disabled Living Foundation*)

Holter valve will be likely to receive the most effective treatment if admitted to the care of the consultant already responsible for the child.

Accidents or sudden illnesses do not always occur when a child is in school or in the care of the parents. For this reason parents may wish to equip their children with something to identify their child's condition such as a diabetic, steroid or anticoagulant card, or a medic-alert bracelet. This enables correct treatment to be started and further information made available at any time of the day or night even though the child may be unconscious and the identity unknown. Parents should be made aware that such services are available.

12. *Mental health* Many people are still very unfamiliar with handicapped people, particularly children, and are not always certain how to react. Consequently, a child may find himself thoroughly rejected and abandoned or over-protected and smothered. For the child to benefit most, some sort of balance must be struck. We have to realize that these children will suffer considerable frustration and stress. They show more behaviour disturbance than normal children which may manifest itself in any of the ways described in Chapter 7. Children who suffer from diseases involving brain dysfunction such as epilepsy and cerebral palsy, show the highest incidence of psychiatric disturbance. This may be particularly marked during adolescence and psychiatric advice needs to be sought. Sexual development may be especially difficult for the handicapped child; sexual appetites will vary as they do with other people, and the handicapped adolescent is equally in need of information and advice, not only about sex but also about genetic counselling. Mentally retarded adolescents may be unable to understand the significance of their actions and some can be embarrassingly precocious indeed; girls may very easily be seduced and become pregnant. There has recently been a great deal of controversy about sterilization of girls thought to be severely handicapped and there are many widely differing views on this question. It is sufficient to say here that the girl's future, her parents' or guardian's future and that of the child she may conceive must all be considered. The whole question of the sexual needs of the handicapped is very controversial and one voluntary organization concerns itself solely with producing literature and information to assist parents and professionals in advising the handicapped.

Mortality is high among the severly handicapped and those with progressive diseases. Consequently, the threat of early death is very real to the child and may be a relatively common occurrence in some schools, particularly residential schools or long-term hospital units. For example, a child with muscular dystrophy is watching his own slow deterioration and may experience the death of a sibling or schoolfriend from the same disease. Death needs to be talked about in a positive way so that it may be accepted and the children need to be allowed to mourn the loss of a friend openly and in their own way.

13. *Record keeping* A continuous daily nursing record should be kept for children needing regular nursing care, particularly where 24-hour cover is involved. A Kardex is easy to refer to and provides a comprehensive history for each child. It is also easily transferred with the medical records if the child moves away, thus providing previous information for the new nurse who can continue the record.

Arrangements in residential schools and hostels Nurses are often appointed in a supervisory capacity to the care of the children during the time when they are not actually in class. There is no doubt that nursing has a place in dealing with certain handicaps but the degree of involvement and necessary training needs defining. Nurses have a tendency to be over-anxious about the prevention of infection and about tidiness and routine, and may consequently run the place in a manner more suitable to a busy surgical ward. Children in residential accommodation need warm mothering and fathering and the creation of an atmosphere as near as possible to that of a good home-life. Children are much more likely to avoid becoming institutionalized and to be able to create homes of their own later on if they are allowed to use their imagination and create something of a personal atmosphere with their own belongings. Participation in local events and activities helps them to feel part of the community and ideally they should develop friendships with children outside the home whose families they may be invited to visit. There should be facilities for a child to return hospitality either himself or, if he is too young, the staff should undertake it on his behalf, encouraging his participation.

Parents may need to be encouraged to visit and facilities for them to stay and carry out parental functions should be available if they have to travel a considerable distance. This is very important in maintaining family ties as indeed are the exchange of letters and telephone calls. Such functions may have to be carried out by the staff for a very young or very severely disabled child. The staff of residential accommodation not associated with the school need to visit the school and discuss the child's work with the teacher as a parent would do. A child ought to be able to bring home his drawings and reports and expect the kind of enthusiasm a parent might express. A good hostel should feel like a happy home and while nursing may be part of such arrangements, it should not dominate the atmosphere. Homes for mentally handicapped children have been sadly lacking in homeliness and indeed is part of the reason why the whole question of nursing and the care of the mentally handicapped is being investigated by a DHSS committee, under the chairmanship of Mrs Peggy Jay.

Social Services Involvement

The 1970 Chronically Sick and Disabled Persons Act requires that local authority social services departments meet the needs of the handicapped. For this reason the social worker will have a large part to play with the handicapped child and his family, whatever the handicap and wherever the child goes to school. Support in the home may include arranging for structural adaptations to be made or special aids such as hoists to be provided or fitted. Families may also have considerable extra expense in providing items such as special clothing and extra laundry and help may be needed in seeking financial assistance.

Help outside the home may extend to arranging holidays, relief for parents during holiday times, as well as transport and travelling facilities, to enable the child to take advantage of local recreation or educational facilities. Sometimes short-term foster care may need to be provided for the relief of parents or if the child is abandoned, long-term fostering arrangements may be required. Information on the sort of help available which can be arranged by the social worker, is contained in the DHSS leaflet HB1 *Help for Handicapped People,* and an up-to-date copy should be kept in the medical room.

Special schools may have a permanent social worker attached to the school and it will be comparatively easy for the nurse to keep in close contact. A nurse working in an ordinary school should ensure that the name, address and telephone number of the social worker responsible for the individual child is entered on the case notes. She should also ensure that she meets and knows the social worker and that regular exchanges are made about the child.

Careers Guidance

Planning for future employment or occupation following school should begin early and the careers officer for special education should be made aware of the child's problems and difficulties at an early stage. This usually happens where children are attending special schools or classes, or having home tuition. However, a child attending ordinary school may easily be missed and not brought to the notice of the careers service at all. This may be very much to the disadvantage of the child or even dangerous to others as, for example, a young person with epilepsy taking a post as a crane driver.

The level of understanding among the general public about handicap is probably fairly low and without sufficient help an adolescent or young adult may find himself in employment where his abilities are under-used, leading to his discontent and depression and to associated emotional problems.

On the open employment market, all employers (with certain exceptions), are at the moment required to employ 3% disabled people as part of their staff. This means finding an employer who can supply work that the young person can undertake satisfactorily in a building that is accessible and suitable to the handicap. Many employers are willing to alter the work load and agree to alterations which the careers officer may suggest. There are a variety of other possibilities depending on the handicap, ability and achievements of the child: university courses or further education may be possible. Sheltered employment which is basically productive and carries ordinary working conditions and expectations may also be arranged. Alternatively, severely disabled people may be placed in diversionary occupations where transport is provided and hours of attendance are shorter.

Medical reports on handicapped children are made by the school doctor on form Y10 and passed to the careers officer. There needs to be close working co-operation between the school health service, the careers service and the Employment Medical Advisory Service which is responsible for advising on the medical aspects of the suitability of employment. EMAS was set up as a result of the Employment Medical Advisory Service Act 1972 and became part of the Health and Safety Executive in 1975. Where practical nursing procedures are involved these may be discussed with nursing advisers from EMAS.

FURTHER READING

Blockley, J. & Miller, G. (1971) Feeding techniques with cerebral-palsied children. *Physiotherapy*, **57**, 7, pp. 300–308.

Bowley, A. H. & Gardner, L. (1972) *The Handicapped Child—Educational and Psychological Guidance for the Organically Handicapped*, 3rd ed. London: Churchill Livingstone.

DHSS Leaflet HB1 (1975) *Help for Handicapped People*. London: HMSO.

Finnie, N. R. (1974) *Handling the Young Cerebral-palsied Child at Home*, 2nd ed. London: Heinemann Medical.

Foott, S. (1976) *The Disabled School Child and Kitchen Sense*. London: Heinemann, for the Disabled Living Foundation.

Forbes, G. (1971) *Clothing for the Handicapped Child*. London: Heinemann, for the Disabled Living Foundation.

Guilliford, R. (1975) *Helping the Handicapped Child at School*. London: National Children's Bureau.

Mandelstem, D. (1977) *Incontinence*, London: Heinemann, for the Disabled Living Foundation.

Oswin, M. (1971) *The Empty Hours—a study of the weekend-life of handicapped children in institutions*. London: Allen Lane.

Ryan, M. (1976) *Feeding Can Be Fun—Advice on Feeding Handicapped Babies and Children*. London: The Spastics Society.

Rudinger, E. (ed.) (1974) *Coping with Disablement*. London: Consumer Association.

Ruston, R. (1977) *Dressing for Disabled People*. London: Disabled Living Foundation. A manual for nurses and others.

Serota & Younghusband Report (1970) *Living with Handicap—Report of a Working Party on Children with Special Needs*. London: National Children's Bureau.

CHILDREN'S BOOKS

Fiction

Fenshaw, E. (1975) *Rachel*. London: Bodley Head. Picture book illustrating how Rachel, who is in a wheelchair, manages to lead a full life, attending the local primary school and joining social activities such as the Brownies. Age 5+ years.

Jessel, C. (1975) *Mark's Wheelchair Adventures*. London: Methuen. Mark has spina bifida and he has to find new friends when his family move house. The new friends include a severely handicapped spastic girl. Age 9+ years.

Larsen, H. (1974) *Don't Forget Tom*. London: Black. Tom is mentally handicapped and his difficulties and relationships with his family are beautifully illustrated. 3+ years.

Southall, I. (1968) *Let the Balloon Go*. London: Methuen. John is left alone for a day and challenges himself to climb a tree in spite of his cerebral palsy. 10+ years.

USEFUL ADDRESSES AND INFORMATION

This is only a small selection of the agencies interested in handicapped children. A very readable and comprehensive list is contained in the *Handbook for Parents with a Handicapped Child* by Judith Stone and Felicity Taylor. A Home and School Council Publication, 1972.

Association for Spina Bifida and Hydrocephalus
30 Devonshire Street
London W1.
Tel: 01 486 6100.

Deals with the welfare of those suffering from spina bifida and hydrocephalus and their families; also promotes researches into causes and treatments.

The British Epilepsy Association
3 Alfred Place
London WC1.
Tel: 01 580 2704.

Publish excellent information leaflets for teachers and nurses.

Cystic Fibrosis Research Trust
5 Blyth Road
Bromley
Kent BR1 3RS.
Tel: 01 464 7211.

Information and advice; also publishes booklets including *Postural Drainage at Home* by Diana Gaskell.

Disabled Living Foundation
346 Kensington High Street
London W14 8NS.
Tel: 01 602 2491.

Permanent exhibition of aids and clothing for the disabled, visits by appointment. Information service on all aspects of disability including other appropriate organizations interested in individual handicaps.

The Family Fund—Joseph Rowntree Memorial Trust
The Secretary
Beverley House
Shipton Road
York YO3 6RB.
Tel: 0904 (York) 29241.

The Rowntree Family Fund (set up by Government in 1972 to help families of children under 16 years).

Friends of the Cheyne Centre for Spastic Children
63 Cheyne Walk
London SW3 5NA.
Tel: 01 352 6740.

Publishes booklets on *Teaching Handicapped Children to Dress and Feed*, written by Cheyne Centre staff. They also run courses and arrange open days at the Centre.

Institute of Mental Subnormality
Lea Castle
Wolverly
Worcestershire DY10 3PP.
Tel: 0562 (Kidderminster) 850251.

Publishes a regular magazine 'Apex' and promotes courses, conferences, workshops and other activities for staff concerned with the mentally subnormal.

Invalid Children's Aid Association
126 Buckingham Palace Road
London SW1W 9SB.
Tel: 01 730 9891.

Concerned with all types of handicap, provides case-work, social services, runs five residential schools and publishes information leaflets and teaching materials.

Medic-alert Foundation
9 Hanover Street
London W1R 9HF.
Tel: 01 499 2261.

Provides 24-hour information service to hospitals, doctors or police, regarding the medical condition of any person wearing a bracelet carrying their insignia.

The National Council for Special Education
1 Wood Street
Stratford on Avon CV37 6JC.
Tel: 0789 5332.

Issues an informative newsletter: probably available from the head-teacher in most special schools.

National Society for the Mentally handicapped
17 Pembridge Square
London W2.
Tel: 01 229 8941.

Only national organization exclusively concerned with the mentally handicapped and their families.

The Spastics Society
12 Park Crescent
London W1.
Tel: 01 636 5020.

Leading organization in the world for the care of children and adults who suffer from cerebral palsy. Also publish useful booklets on the management of spastics, courses and conferences. Extensive training programmes arranged for professional staff dealing with handicap.

SPOD (Committee on Sexual Problems for the Disabled)
49 Victoria Street
London SW1.
Tel: 01 222 6067.

Associated with the National Fund for Research into crippling diseases. Publishes helpful leaflets and organizes seminars for professional staff dealing with the handicapped. Deals with all aspects of sexual problems of the disabled.

Voluntary Council for Handicapped Children
National Children's Bureau
8 Wakeley Street
London EC1V 7QE.
Tel: 01 278 9441.

Set up under National Children's Bureau, offers help and advice on all aspects of handicap to parents and professionals.

Discussion Topics

1. You have a handicapped child in an ordinary school and notice he is not using appliances which have been issued. Consider any possible reasons and the action you would take in each case.

2. You receive a message that a child whose home is in your area but who attends a residential school 100 miles away, requires regular home visiting during the holiday. You have no other information. What would you do?

3. The doctor has issued a new prescription increasing the dosage of an anti-convulsant drug. What information does the teacher need and how are the unused drugs from the last prescription to be treated?

4. You are a visiting nurse in an ordinary primary school. You accidentally hear that the head teacher is considering admitting a spina bifida child in a wheelchair. Would this be of concern to you and what action might you take?

5. A locum general practitioner is sent to carry out a school medical examination. He suspects one child to be very backward and in need of special education but is unsure of the procedure and asks your advice. How would you assist him?

6. A handicapped child requiring a good deal of assistance from care staff and nurses is slowly gaining more confidence and becoming less dependent. Consider ways in which you might ensure that (1) the child does not regress in the holidays and (2) the whole family enjoy the holiday.

9
Nursing Surveys, Clinics and Visiting

Routine Health Check

Normally the school nurse sees every child in the school once a year. This is essentially a screening exercise and gives a person with medical knowledge an opportunity to make an assessment of the child's health; at present it varies from a cursory look at the child to a more detailed examination, depending on the time available, the training of the nurse and the expectations of the medical and senior nursing staff. The importance of this examination will undoubtedly increase as selective medicals become generally accepted. The aim of these examinations is to discover any conditions which should be brought to the attention of the doctor or dentist.

Children due for routine or selective medical examinations should have their screening procedures completed before the examination. This may be done at separate sessions or combined with the medical examination as described in Chapter 4.

Routine screening generally includes measurement of height, weight, head circumference (only necessary at entry), immunization state, vision, hearing and general observation of the child's behaviour. Some doctors like to include a urine sample as there is some evidence that bacteriuria is common in school children[1]. Children not having a selective medical in addition to the annual screening should have the benefit of a longer time for discussion with the nurse and more extensive general observation by her. These examinations also provide the nurse with opportunities for individual health education. The organization of the health check and the individual observations required will be influenced by the previous history and the doctor's examination comments together with the age, development and ethnic origin of the child.

Young children By far the most common illnesses in the young child's life are respiratory diseases and associated chronic infections of the throat and ears, and any health check needs to take account of the frequency of these, the treatment the child received and any consequences likely to result, hearing loss, for example. Parents who are working or who are not very adept at managing problems may not understand how to care for the child properly during illness. Their children return to school in a low state and are often chronically 'below par'. Such parents and their children can often be helped by the district nurse or school nurse visiting during illness to encourage and teach the mother. They also need to understand that infections in childhood are part of the process by which children develop natural immunity and that constant requests to the doctor to prescribe antibiotics for minor infections is not always in the child's interests.

Other very common occurrences during the primary years include infectious and contagious diseases, dental caries, bed-wetting and accidents. Non-accidental injury may also be seen in the primary school and this needs immediate medical consultation and follow-up by the social services. Common chronic conditions usually already identified include asthmas and epilepsy.

Adolescence This begins at various ages, usually $10\frac{1}{2}$ to 13 years in girls, and $12\frac{1}{2}$ to 15 years in boys, which means that in a class of children in the 10 to 15 age range, children of the same age may be entirely different in their physical and emotional maturity. Once children have reached the age of puberty, they need to be increasingly encouraged to start making their own decisions and to discipline and organize their lives. This helps them to transfer more easily from the school routine to the adult life and freedom of college, university or work. Decisions about health will also be part of that life and therefore they should be encouraged as far as possible to seek consultation with the doctor and nurse rather than to be subjected to it. They are unlikely to be forthcoming during an unwilling interview which will probably not prove beneficial to anyone. Prevention of illness is increasingly possible through screening and early use of health services and therefore ways must be found through the school health education system and the organization of the school health service to encourage consultation and use of the service.

Adolescents appear to have a surprisingly high record of physical illness which often prevents them attending school. A recent survey[2] suggested that the most common complaints are respiratory diseases, headaches, menstrual pains, acne, asthma and wheezy bronchitis. Colds, sore throats and accidents are very common and some 1% of 16-year-olds are still bed-wetting. Admission to hospital is usually for tonsilitis and appendicitis.

Nurses who are employed full-time in secondary schools are likely to be in a position to deal with some of these complaints and perhaps reduce absenteeism and some of the work-load on hospital casualty departments and family practitioners. Advice sought for apparently minor complaints also provides the nurse with opportunities for individual health education and screening for height, weight and vision (particularly important at puberty).

Adolescence may be a difficult time for some children. Sexually mature adolescents may be experiencing all the emotional upheavals of dating the opposite sex and some may be sexually active with either one or more partners. The incidence of pregnancy among schoolgirls is rising; indeed the current estimate is around 5000 per year[3]. The social and health consequences for these girls are considerable and every effort needs to be made to avoid this situation by giving guidance and, if necessary, contraceptive advice. Boys are equally in need of advice and too often this aspect of their education is neglected. The school nurse may or may not be equipped to do this, depending on her experience and agreed role in the school. However, she should know who to refer to and also be sufficiently at ease to discover the problem initially and gain the adolescent's consent to referral. Some school nurses may have taken a family planning and counselling course and may also work in the local adolescent advisory clinic in which case referral is relatively easy.

Ethnic origins Nurses working in schools where there are children from various ethnic groups need to familiarize themselves with their background and cultures. This helps them to understand the reasoning behind the parents' way of life and the kinds of conflict experienced by children educated in an English school and living in a home where the language and way of life bears no relationship to the school situation.

Certain illnesses are more likely to occur in children[4] of some ethnic groups and health checks should take this into account. Nurses working with such children would be well advised to study these in some depth.

Rickets This disease results from lack of vitamin D and is likely to present in the 9 to 16-year-old age group; indeed, some surveys[5] have suggested that 20 to 30% of Indian and Pakistani children, particularly girls at puberty, are likely to be affected. Children with rickets generally look undernourished and often complain of tiredness and limb pains, or they may have difficulty in running. Where cases are confirmed, the whole family should be examined.

Anaemia Iron deficiency anaemia may occur in children whose parents have difficulty in obtaining their national foods or adapting English substitutes. Sickle cell anaemia is quite common in Negro children who may complain of limb and joint pains, severe abdominal pains and fever. Where cases are confirmed the children must avoid over-tiredness, infections and over-exposure to the elements.

Thalassaemia This occurs in children from Mediterranean countries and India; it is usually progressive from birth.

Tuberculosis This disease is very common among new immigrants[6], particularly those from the Indian subcontinent, Africa, the West Indies and Ireland. The advantages of BCG protection need to be explained and offered as soon as possible (see p. 142).

Malaria This may occur in children from tropical or subtropical regions, or in those who have recently visited a malarial country without taking preventive drug treatment.

Intestinal worms Round worms and hook worms may be found among children who have recently arrived in this country; those most often infested are usually from Asia. Worms are generally picked up by walking barefoot on ground contaminated by faeces containing the eggs; therefore, good sanitation is an important aspect of prevention. Worms cause anaemia and diagnosis is confirmed when the eggs are found in the stools.

Health Check Preparation
Arrangements should as usual be made with the head teacher in good time. The selection of children will depend on their individual needs and availability. The school time-table will show which children will be absent for classes such as swimming and physical education. Children do not have to undress for nursing checks and therefore it is unnecessary to have written parental consent. However, parents should know the purpose of these surveys and information should be contained in the school information booklet and also given to parents at parent–teacher association meetings. The children should understand why they are being taken from the class-room and it is advisable to fetch only a few children at a time, firstly because they should lose as little time as possible from their lessons, and secondly because the greater number there are the less easy they are to control. The nurse's task is made very much easier if a school helper, member of staff or monitor organizes the children, fetches them to and from class and gives general assistance to the nurse. On the other hand, fetching the children herself gives the nurse an opportunity to visit the class-room, to see the children at work and to see whether those who should wear glasses, hearing aids and other appliances are doing so. The school register will reveal which children are absent and show the frequency of absenteeism, particularly for illness. Prolonged discussion with the class teacher will probably be more appropriate in the staff room or at break times.

In Chapter 7 I outlined the importance of noting the child's progress and reactions at school. Consequently, exchange of such information between teacher and nurse is essential if the child is to be seen in total context of his life in school. Any of the following arising from such discussion should be regarded as matters for concern:

1. Frequent absence from school, particularly when sickness is given as the reason.

2. Poor concentration, restlessness or fidgeting; alternatively, day-dreaming or having blank spells.
3. Quarrelling or bullying, or destruction of personal belongings or school property.
4. Lack of friends or solitariness, being irritable, whining or miserable.
5. Mannerisms such as thumb-sucking or nail-biting and twitches or tics.
6. Timidity, fussiness and lying or stealing.
7. Incontinence or soiling, constant complaints of headaches or pains, and visible skin rashes.
8. Speech or learning problems.

Such complaints should be noted in the medical record and brought to the doctor's attention.

The survey should be carried out in the medical room or in accommodation allocated for the purpose. Each child should be seen individually though very' young children often like their friends to be present to give them confidence and make them more relaxed. The child's general demeanour and behaviour while waiting should be noted.

To put the child at ease it is advisable to start with practical screening procedures with which the child can participate and then gradually proceed to more personal details. Each nurse will find a preferred routine which may vary according to the age of the child. The nurse who has experience will immediately put the child at ease, encouraging the child to talk—Does he like school? Who are his friends? Which lessons does he like? What reading book is he using? What games does he play?—all of which not only puts the child at ease but supplies a good deal of useful information to the nurse. The name of any school child new to the district and having siblings under five years of age should be notified to the health visitor.

Posture and limbs Notice the child's gait on entering the room and the standing and sitting posture; general slouching; round shoulders; protruding shoulder-blades; knock-knees; bow-legs or flat feet are all worthy of the attention of the doctor and physical education teacher.

Height and weight Measurements of height and weight were for a time unfashionable in schools. However, they have now resumed their former importance as indicators of the child's nutritional state and of his growth and development. Measurements should be accurate and are charted on the Tanner and Whitehouse Height and Weight Standard Charts which indicate the average for the child's age and the accepted normal range (see Fig. 22). Instructions for accurate use are also printed on the charts. The lines on the chart represent 'centiles' within which you would expect measurements to fall. Normally a child will continue to grow along the line she starts on. For example, the child who starts on the 10th centile should be discussed with the doctor if marked deviations from that line occur: she may have some developmental abnormality though ethnic group and parental build must be taken into account. Nutrition may need serious consideration in both home and school; indeed these charts are the most likely early indication of obesity. Neglect cannot be ruled out and these records have been used as additional evidence at court proceedings for cases of child abuse.

The scales should be checked and serviced regularly to see that they are properly balanced and each child should wear the amount of clothing agreed with the doctor. It is usual to weigh an average set of the clothing and subtract this from the weight of each child.

Height measures should preferably be fixed to the wall and for accurate readings a right-angled block of wood or head-piece should be used. The most satisfactory height measure is the Harpenden Stadiometer pictured in use (Fig. 23). The use of pencils, rulers and flimsy insecure head-pieces renders the exercise inaccurate and the resulting chart may even reveal that the child is shrinking!

To chart the measurements, a transparent ruler should be used. Find the child's age along the bottom line and the height or weight along the vertical line and mark the place where the two meet. Each mark should be joined to the last one to form a growth graph and present a picture of the child's progress.

Eyes Examine the eyes for any sign of squint or abnormality of shape or size; conjunctivitis or blepharitis should be noted and the child referred for treatment. Vision should be screened as required (see Chapter 5).

Hearing Check that the hearing has been screened. Listen to the speech and conversation for any indications of hearing defect as suggested in Chapter 6. Any earaches, discharge or excessive wax should be referred for treatment.

Hair and scalp The hair and scalp are examined for infestation and dandruff. Part the hair with the hands or a comb and inspect the roots. Nits (eggs of the head-louse) are generally seen within 1 cm of the scalp and are to be found on the front of the head on boys, and on the sides and behind the ears in girls (see p. 148). When scraped with a comb, dandruff will flake away but nits cling firmly to the hair and cannot be removed. Any evidence of infestation must be treated as described on p. 148. Bald patches are sometimes seen particularly in West Indian children whose hair has been tightly plaited though the cause may, of course, be ringworm; diagnosis can be confirmed by the use of a Wood's glass.

Throat, teeth and abdomen Examine the throat for inflammation and note any complaints of tonsillitis or repeated sore throats. Record any evidence of enlarged glands. While examining the throat, look closely at the condition of the teeth. Gingivitis is extremely common in school children and any bleeding or inflammation of the gums needs investigation by the dental service. Ask the child how often he is taken to the dentist either by his parents or through the school dental service. There may also be pain from neglected decay, erupting

Name.. Date of Birth .... Reg. No. ....

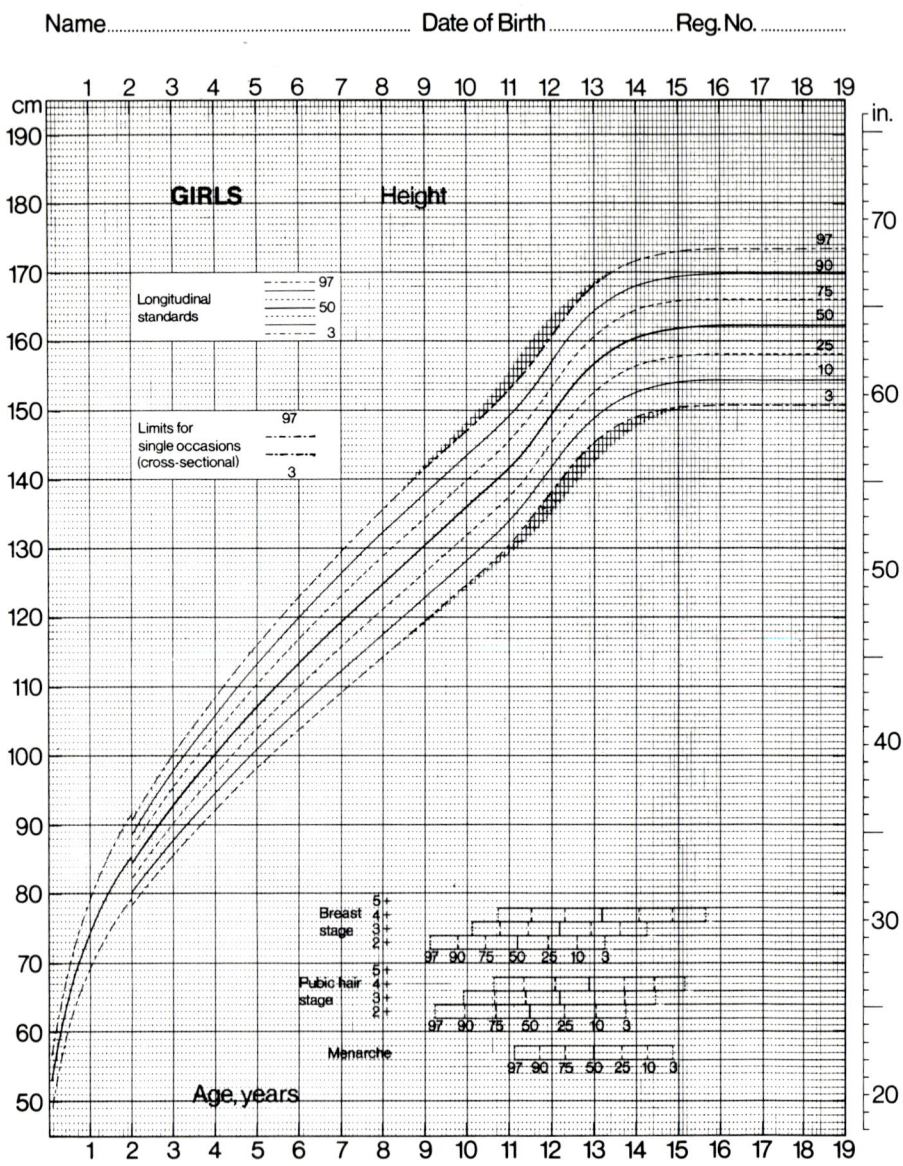

Fig. 22. *Tanner and Whitehouse Standard Height and Weight Chart for girls (similar chart appropriate for boys available). (Creaseys)*

Name .... Date of Birth .... Reg. No. ....

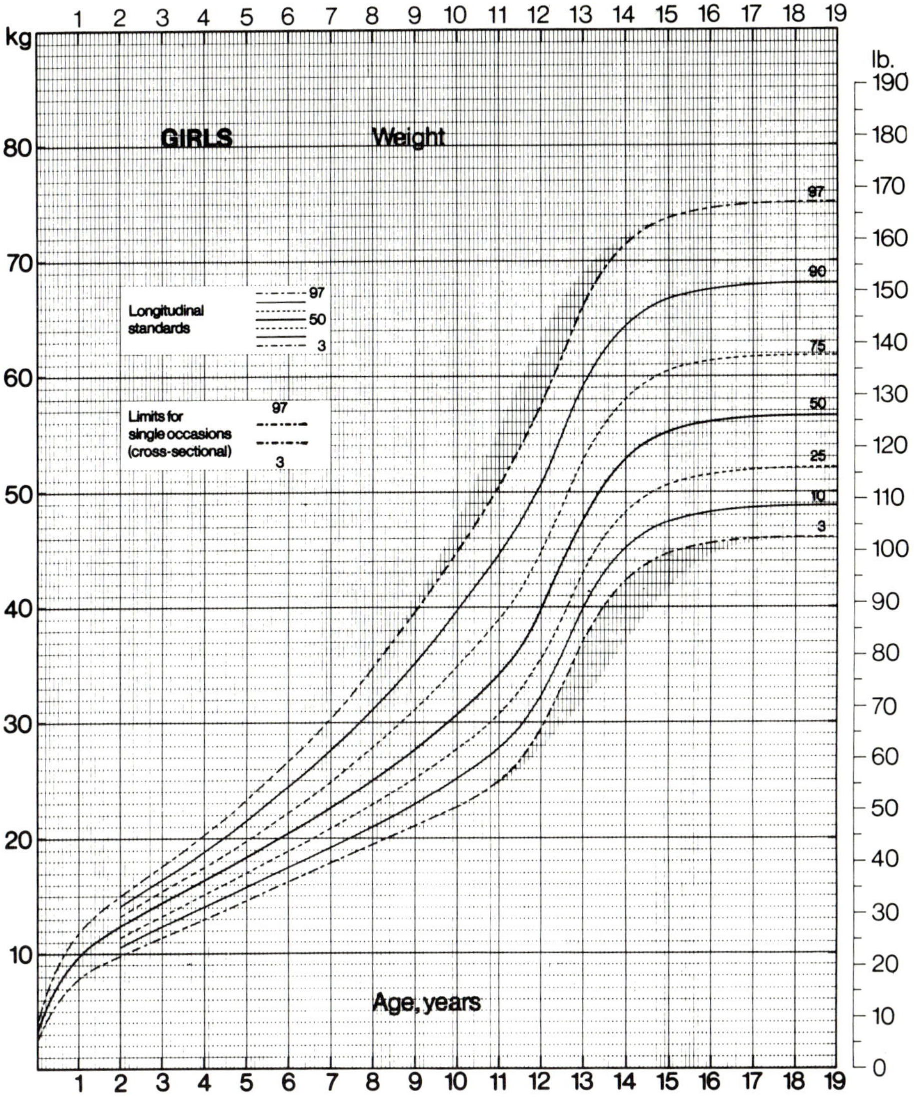
GIRLS
Weight
kg
lb.
Longitudinal standards
97
50
3
Limits for single occasions (cross-sectional)
97
3
97
90
75
50
25
10
3
Age, years
1 2 3 4 5 6 7 8 9 10 11 12 13 14 15 16 17 18 19
10 20 30 40 50 60 70 80
0 10 20 30 40 50 60 70 80 90 100 110 120 130 140 150 160 170 180 190

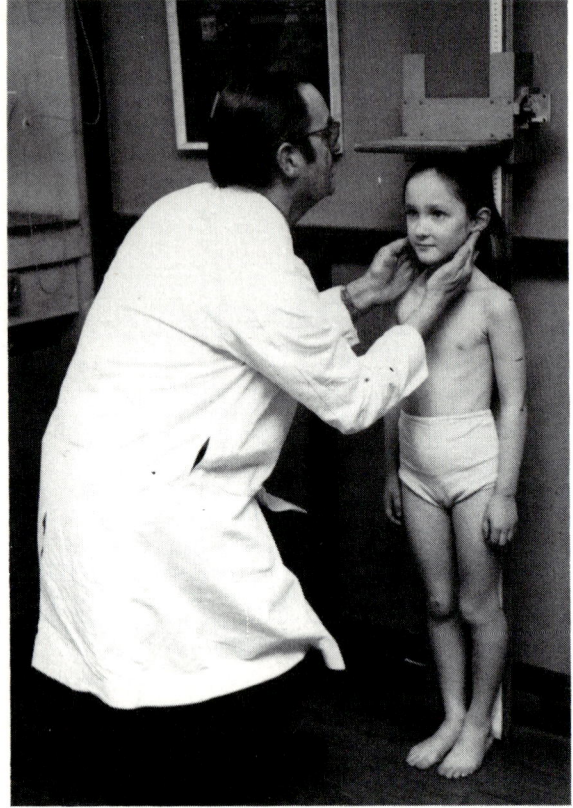

Fig. 23. Harpenden Stadiometer in use. Notice tall stance and positioning of the child. (Institute of Child Health)

wisdom teeth or following deep fillings; badly stained teeth and 'bad breath' also need attention.

Take the opportunity to reinforce the school dental policy on oral hygiene. This may be an appropriate time to discuss diet—does the child have a proper breakfast before coming to school or is he given pocket money to buy something on the way, which may turn out to be sweets? does he eat school meals?—this information, if suspect, can be checked with the school meals personnel. In some large schools bullying by aggressive children sometimes extends to preventing timid shy children from eating. Frequently, complaints of upset tummies or pains are the result of poor diet and constipation.

Nose and lungs Observe any catarrh, colds or sneezing and question the child about their duration and frequency; notice any nasal speech. Question the child about breathlessness or wheezing, including when and how it occurs and record any school absences for bronchitis or chest complaints.

Skin and feet The child should not be undressed but the exposed parts may be examined for impetigo, abscesses, boils, carbuncles, eczema or insect bites. The general condition of the feet should be noted; cramped toes may indicate that shoes or socks are too small, and toe-nails may be incorrectly cared for, thereby predisposing to future foot deformities. Shoes and socks should be removed and the feet inspected for varrucae or athlete's foot (nursing treatment of contagious disease described on pp. 147–54).

Sexual maturation The stage of sexual maturation should be noted, i.e. girl's body, bust, date of commencement of periods; boy's body and voice maturation. Occasionally, a child may have caught a venereal disease and any complaint of vaginal discharges, itching, or sores on the vagina or penis should be referred to the doctor. Complaints of dry scaly skin and excessive loss of hair when combing, combined with raised temperature, swollen glands and spots in the mouth and genitals may indicate secondary syphilis which has been known to present in a school child.

General observation The child's personal hygiene and general care should be noted and the state and appropriateness of his clothing which may indicate a great deal about the parents' attitudes, or indeed the activities of the last class. For example, further investigations might be needed into the reasons for a child wearing a summer dress on a cold winter's day. Stains on the clothing may be present for all sorts of innocent reasons or they may be present as a result of undesirable activities, such as glue sniffing.

The present immunization state should be recorded. Inquire about any attendances to the family practitioner or hospital casualty department and record them with the reasons. Any medicines being taken should be noted and, if they are being brought to school, enquiries should be made as to the arrangements for administration and safe-keeping. Finally, any children with employment certificates should be observed for tiredness or absence from school. A nurse who is trusted by the children and consulted by them will not have to spend long periods of time on these surveys as much of the information will be already known to her from her day to day contact with the staff and children.

Action

Where no further action is required the child should be told that he is well and healthy and asked to return to the class-room. If further investigation is needed, explain this to the child and also what steps you are taking to discuss this with the parents. Some aspects of personal hygiene, care of the teeth or diet may need discussion, preferably backed up with written information. The nurse may wish to pursue this individually by seeing the child again or where a class of children present with similar health education needs, this might be discussed with the teacher and arrangements made to include this in the teaching programme. Problems which call for discussion with the doctor or dentist should be dealt with as soon as possible. Poorly-clad or neglected children may need to be discussed with the social worker or the educations welfare service, as appropriate.

Recording and record checks A note of the survey and any special observations should be made on the child's medical record. Special nursing documentation may be available for the purpose, otherwise it should be entered on the M.10 (school medical record). Regular record checks are also needed to follow up the results of any further investigations suggested.

Selective Surveys

Surveys must be carried out selectively for particular reasons. Where there is a reasonably high incidence of contagious disease, hygiene inspections of hair, hands and feet may be carried out routinely at the beginning of term. Should contagious or infectious disease be confirmed in the school during the term, contacts need special inspection for suspicious symptoms, depending on the disease in question. When a doctor's certificate is not obtainable, surveys may include inspection of children 24 to 48 hours before departure on a school journey. This is to confirm that all treatment and injections recommended by the doctor have been completed (see p. 47) and that there are no symptoms of infectious disease in any member of the party. Any suspicious symptoms should be confirmed by a doctor and the child excluded. This can be very stressful and upsetting for the child, parent and the whole school party, and sometimes for the nurse who may be seen as the culprit. However, adequate treatment is ensured if the child stays at home and the rest of the party are more likely to enjoy their trip.

Selective surveys are generally conducted with groups of about six to ten children, usually seen together and preferably in the medical room. It is advisable to have a school helper or auxiliary to organize the children, fetching them from the class-room and keeping order as they queue up. It is usually less disruptive to see the noisy children first. This also gives the shyer children a chance to relax. The helper instructs them to open their collars, roll back sleeves and remove shoes and socks, according to the reason for inspection. However, it is unlikely that one nurse and one auxiliary will be able to inspect the whole school in one day. This means, particularly for head inspection, that undiscovered infectious children may infect the children already seen. A more satisfactory method has proved to be groups of nurses or trained auxiliaries inspecting the whole school in one day. The nurse should visit the school early on the following morning to inspect any children absent on the previous day and at the same time check that any child found to be infectious on the previous day has in fact received treatment. Inspection for contagious disease should be carried out as follows:

Hair	inspect for nits and lice (see p. 127).
Neck	inspect for swollen glands, boils or rash, impetigo, scabs or vesicles.
Fingers, Nails, Hands and Wrists	inspect the fingers and nails for warts, ringworm, severe nail-biting, and evidence of scabies between the fingers or on the wrists or backs of the hands. Complaints of itching may indicate unseen patches of scabies on the trunk.
Feet	inspect the feet for plantar warts, and between the toes, particularly the fourth and fifth toes for ringworm (athlete's foot).

Visiting the class-room Time should be allowed to visit the class-rooms at intervals. This can normally be fitted in with occasions when the nurse may fetch the children from class or following surveys when some matter needs to be discussed with the teacher. This provides an opportunity to observe the children in class and to get the feel of the class-room atmosphere, whilst the children see the nurse as part of the school community. It is also an opportunity to see something of the methods of education in the school and to observe the children's work, subsequently using these observations to initiate conversation with a child or develop some individual health teaching.

Primary school children do a lot of colourful project work generally displayed on the walls. This not only indicates the topics that the children are interested in and are learning about, but also shows how they interpret the world and their feelings about it; occasionally, it blatantly displays a vision defect which has been missed. Occasions like school plays and parties give added opportunities for getting to know the children and their parents.

School clinics The doctor's role in school clinics has already been described on p. 51. Nursing activities may also be carried out for school children either in the local health centre, child health clinic or in the school itself.

Minor ailments such as more serious cuts or lacerations, septic sores, skin diseases and eye and ear infections are often dealt with at special sessions, ranging in length and frequency from one hour or more daily to an hour or less three times per week. Many nurses and doctors question the need for these sessions although a large number of children do attend accident and emergency departments and family practitioners for minor ailments. Most parents carry out much of this sort of minor nursing treatment for their children and many less capable mothers can also manage this once they have been taught by a sympathetic nurse. A lone working parent may not be able to cope, and neglected children certainly need some provision for this sort of care. Where there is a full-time school nurse it becomes part of her first-aid activities and there is no difficulty in arranging this during breaktimes.

Home visiting Home visits may be necessary for a number of reasons. The parents may not have attended the medical examination or seemed to have had difficulty in understanding some part of the discussion. It may be necessary to explain or reinforce some health aspect arising from either the medical or the nursing survey. Where children travel considerable distances to school and the school health services are administered by different area health authorities, nurses must ask their colleagues in the home area to visit the child's home on their behalf and to report back.

Generally, visits should only be undertaken by nursing staff if nursing expertise or background knowledge is required. Follow-up of failed appointments and visits in connection with social problems are undertaken by education, welfare and social service staff. There may be overlap and variations throughout the country, depending on the staffing arrangement of the various departments.

Every visit should have a definite purpose and the nurse should know clearly what she hopes to achieve, anticipate any difficulties which may arise, such as language barriers, in which case it may be necessary to ensure that an interpreter can be present. Generally less time is wasted if appointments can be made in advance unless they are unlikely to be understood or kept.

Good home visiting is an art in itself which improves with experience and results from sensitive instinct combined with observance of some basic principles. It should be remembered that a nurse has no right of entry into a home and only has access by courtesy and invitation of the family. This is more likely to happen if the nurse:

1. presents a pleasant, acceptable and professional image, attired in a fashion unlikely to embarrass the family or make them feel awkward;
2. has an easy manner encouraging the family to talk by prompting conversation rather than questioning;
3. observes social practices such as tea-drinking with sensitivity, understanding the circumstances in which to accept or decline;
4. observes the confidentiality of information given to her by the family, only revealing it with their consent (other than in exceptional circumstances where failure to do so might have adverse results for the child, for example non-accidental injury).

The family have no obligation to follow advice given and are only likely to do so because they see the advantage to themselves or to the child. This is health education in a one-to-one situation but the principle of changing attitudes (as described in Chapter 11) equally applies.

A note of the home visit should be entered on the medical record. The reason for the visit should be clearly stated and also whether this was accomplished. It may not be possible to know immediately whether action will result from a visit in which case a careful note needs to be made and a follow-up visit planned.

REFERENCES

1. Edward, B. et al. (1975) Screening methods for covert bacteriuria in schoolgirls. *Br. med.J.* **ii**, pp. 463–467.
2. Fogelman, K. (ed.) (1976) *Britain's Sixteen Year Olds*. London: National Children's Bureau.
3. Editorial (1976) Schoolgirl pregnancies. *Br. med.J.* **ii**, p. 545.
4. Goel, K. M. (1976) Diseases of immigrant children. *Nursing Mirror* **142**, *16*, pp. 55–57.
5. Ford, J. A. (1970) Rickets and Osteomalacia. *Nursing Times* **70**, *2*, pp. 49–50.
6. Report from Br. Thoracic & Tuberculosis Association. (1975) *Tuberculosis among immigrants*, related to length of residence in England and Wales. *Br. med J.* **iii**, pp. 698–699.

FURTHER READING

Darke, S. J. & Stephen, J. M. L. (1976) *Vitamin D Deficiency and Osteomalacia*. London: DHSS, HMSO.

Illingworth, R. S. (1974) *The Child at School*, Oxford: Blackwell Scientific.

Mahoney, E. A., Verdisco, L. & Shortridge, L. (1976) *How to Collect and Record a Health History*. Philadelphia: Lippincott. Distributed by Blackwell Scientific.

Nemir, A. (1970) *The School Health Programme*. Eastbourne: Saunders. A textbook for teachers, school nurses, school administrators.

Pringle, M. K. (1974) *The Needs of Children*. London: Hutchinson, for the National Children's Bureau.

Thurmott, P. (1976) *Health and the School*. London: Royal College of Nursing. An exploratory survey of the school nursing service in an English county.

CHILDREN'S BOOKS

Non-Fiction

Showers, P. (1969) *How Many Teeth*. London: Black.

Fiction

Rockwell, H. (1975) *My Dentist*. London: Hamish Hamilton. Picture book illustrating dental equipment and procedure very well. —5 years.

Starter series. (1971) *Teeth*. London: MacDonald. Picture book illustrating teeth, toothache and visit to the dentist. 3+ years.

Whitney, A. M. (1971) *Just Awful*. London: W. Work. James cuts his finger and dreads going to the school nurse until he finds she is not so bad after all. 5+ years.

USEFUL ADDRESSES AND INFORMATION

Commission for Racial Equality
(Previously known as Community Relations Commission)
15–16 Bedford Street
London WC2E QHX.
Tel: 01 836 3545.

Produces information booklets on all aspects of immigrant problems. Runs seminars on relevant topics, including particular health problems. Will give advice and information as to where to obtain assistance locally.

National Children's Bureau
8 Wakeley Street
London EC1.
Tel: 01 278 9441.

Information, research and short training courses on all aspects of health and social welfare of children.

Discussion Topics

1. What factors in a school would indicate that selective surveys for contagious diseases might be adopted routinely? Would you accept this as a long-term situation (see Chapter 11).

2. A suspected polio outbreak has meant that all school nursing staff have been so involved in the immunization programme that insufficient time is left to complete the yearly nursing sensory screening check. How would you select the children most in need of screening?

3. You take up a post as school nurse in a secondary school where there have recently been several schoolgirl pregnancies. You enquire as to what action is being taken to prevent this situation in the future and to deal with the present problem. You are told that this is not your concern. Discuss.

3. You are invited to the end of term sports and work exhibition. Would you accept and if so why, and what would you be particularly interested in?

4. You do a home visit and the mother does not invite you in but talks to you on the doorstep. Consider possible reasons for this and how you might follow up the visit.

5. The head teacher is complaining because so many children are missing several lessons, allegedly because they are attending the accident and emergency departments. Discuss how you might investigate the situation (with reference to Chapters 2 and 12) and the sort of solutions which might be considered.

10

Infectious and Contagious Diseases

The responsibility for control of infectious diseases rests with the environmental health department of the local authority to whom medical advice is usually given by the proper officer (medical officer for environmental health). Local arrangements for control in school vary considerably and the responsibility may be shared between the area specialist in community medicine (child health) and the medical officer for environmental health.

Children are prone to infectious diseases and any nurse working in school should be familiar with the signs and symptoms for early identification, the incubation periods and method of spread and the preventive action to take, both for infectious diseases and contagious diseases common in schools. No attempt is made here to describe in detail individual diseases as there are many excellent well-illustrated books on the market and for the school nurse the section on communicable diseases contained in the *Handbook of School Health*[1] could hardly be bettered.

INFECTIOUS DISEASES

Certain diseases are carefully monitored in Britain by the DHSS and internationally by the World Health Organization so that immediate measures to prevent further outbreaks may be instituted. These diseases are listed by the DHSS as notifiable and doctors are paid a small fee to notify cases to the medical officer for environmental health who sends a weekly return to the DHSS. Alterations may be made at government level as in 1976 when two cases of lassa fever were confirmed and this was subsequently added to the list. Local additions may be made by the medical officer for environmental health as he thinks fit. The present national list is as follows:

Acute encephalitis.	Measles.
Acute meningitis.	Paratyphoid fever.
Acute poliomyelitis.	Plague.
Anthrax.	Rabies.
Cholera.	Relapsing fever.
Diphtheria.	Scarlet fever.
Dysentery (amoebic and bacillary).	Smallpox.
Food poisoning.	Tetanus.
Infective jaundice.	Tuberculosis.
Lassa fever.	Typhoid fever.
Leprosy.	Typhus.
Leptospirosis.	Whooping cough.
Malaria.	Yellow fever.

Many of these are now, fortunately, extremely rare and certainly unlikely to be seen in school. The most common infectious diseases among the children are likely to be chickenpox, measles and mumps.

The DHSS documents on the Control of Communicable Disease in Schools[2] recommend that there should be clear local procedures for notification of children absent from school for infectious disease. These procedures together with a chart indicating the action to be taken and the recommended exclusion times in suspected cases should be available in every school and known to the school health team and the teachers. Nursing responsibilities in connection with infectious disease should include:

1. Prevention and protection.
2. Identification.
3. Contact tracing and action in school.
4. Contact tracing and action in the home.
5. Isolation nursing in residential units.
6. Action on return to school.

Prevention and Protection

This is achieved in three ways

1. Clean environment.
2. Screening of school staff.
3. Immunity—natural and artificial.

Clean environment Infection is easily picked up and transferred in any large group of people. The school environment should be such that the risks are minimized as much as possible, as well as providing an example for children to follow at home. The nurse and the doctor need to encourage good health practice and point out deficiencies to the teachers and administrators. Attention should be paid to the following points:

   a. Provision of adequate building, no overcrowding, stuffy rooms, plenty of fresh air, sufficient toilets and hand-basins with adequate provision of toilet paper, soap and paper towels, or warm-air driers. Roller towels are not satisfactory

   b. General state of cleanliness of whole school, particularly toilets, hand-basins, showers and changing rooms with satisfactory rubbish disposal, clean play-grounds free of animal excreta.

   c. School organization should encourage good personal hygiene with hand-washing before meals and after visiting the toilet.

   d. State of repair and replacement of blocked drains, taps and faulty toilets.

   e. Storage and serving of food and disposal of left-overs.

   f. Arrangements for keeping and caring for school pets and laboratory animals, birds and insects.

Screening of school staff All staff working in schools should have a medical examination and a chest X-ray before being employed and these should be repeated as necessary. Rubella vaccine should also be offered to all female staff if they have not already been protected. Some education authorities have their own occupational health service and this function is carried out by them for teachers, food handlers and other educational staff. The NHS occupational health service will perform these duties with respect to school doctors and nurses.

Food handlers are particularly important as careless or no handwashing following visits to the toilet, continuing to handle food while suffering from diarrhoea or an open hand lesion may easily cause an outbreak of infection. Supervisors are usually careful to see that staff have good hygiene teaching, and, if infectious, they are given alternative work or permission to stay at home, as appropriate. School meals staff with bowel infections are not normally allowed to return until they have three negative stool specimens. Where poor practice is observed in school this should be brought to the attention of the supervisor.

Staff also need protection and because of the risk to a newly-conceived fetus all female staff in the school should be warned when a case of rubella is reported. If they have not been vaccinated they may ask for transfer to alternative duties or visit the doctor for a gammaglobulin injection.

Immunity Antibodies defend the body against infection and are transferred before birth to the fetus via the placenta and are acquired during the early childhood months from breast milk. Gradually the child starts developing *natural* immunity through contact with common infections causing colds and coughs. The healthy child has sufficient resources to produce antibodies which may defend the body for a period of time or throughout life. Only when infections are known to be sufficiently severe to cause permanent handicap or death should medication or *artificial* immunity be considered. Either small doses of live viruses may be injected into the body to produce natural immunity or artificial antibodies may be administered. As the incidence of a particular disease falls, two things happen:

a. The body has less opportunity to acquire a natural immunity as there is no contact with the disease. This means that until the disease is eradicated world-wide, the unprotected unimmunized person is extremely vulnerable in another country with higher incidence.
b. As a disease becomes eradicated, the side effects of immunization will probably cause more illnesses than the disease itself. This has the effect of deterring people from being immunized. Once the level of protection in the country falls very low, we run the risk of a major outbreak if a carrier enters the country.

The DHSS monitor infectious diseases closely through the notification system. These notifications are monitored world-wide by the World Health Organization and when, as in the case of smallpox, the disease is felt to be eradicated, vaccination is no longer required. Immunization begins in the pre-school years. The national scheme laid down by the DHSS is outlined in Table 2. The actual timing schedules of vaccinations vary locally, according to the

Table 2. Scheme for immunization laid down by the DHSS

Age (years)	Disease	Dose	
0–1	Diphtheria	3	
	Tetanus	3	
	Whooping cough	3	
	Poliomyelitis	3	
1–2	Measles vaccine		
5	Diphtheria	Booster	
	Tetanus	Booster	
	Poliomyelitis	Booster	
10–13	BCG vaccine*	For tuberculine negative school children	
11–13 (girls only)	Rubella	Acceptance appears better at 11 years	
15–19 (or school-leaving)	Tetanus	Booster	
	Poliomyelitis	Booster	

* Tuberculosis has a higher incidence in certain ethnic groups such as Irish or Asian peoples., Some areas with large populations of these groups are adopting policies of giving BCG at birth or at 5 years on school entry.

judgement of the medical staff. The health authority usually issue a printed schedule card for the mother to keep when the programme is commenced and this is signed each time another injection is given. This should, if possible, be kept up in school so that the young adult has a personal record to keep for future reference.

The 0 to 5 year schedule should be completed before school entry or entry to play-group or nursery school. Groups are much more likely to be sources of infection for a young child, particularly for measles which is still a common occurrence. Mothers need to be discouraged from starting unprotected children in group activities during outbreaks of measles or worse still arranging for the child to have measles vaccination and immediately exposing him to the additional infection.

Where there is a low up-take of immunization and there are many mobile families it may be useful to discuss the problem with the head teachers concerned, and make arrangements for immunization to be discussed with the parents at their interview with the head before school entry. This will identify children unknown to the health visitor who require pre-school follow-up. This is also a good time to establish where the mother may be contacted if the child is ill although this information needs to be regularly up-dated.

At one time all immunization and vaccination procedures were carried out by the doctor. However, in recent years, some doctors have delegated this responsibility to nurses. The DHSS recognize this and advise that all areas should have a policy regarding the nurse's role. Such policies should clearly define the injections which may be given by the nurse, and the legal responsibilities of the doctor, nurse and the area health authority. Immunization and vaccination does have an element of risk for a child, particularly in certain circumstances, and, consequently, an nurse undertaking immunization should ensure that she is aware of the area health authority policy and that she is fully conversant with the procedure, the contraindications to the injections she has agreed to administer and the action to take in cases of anaphylactic shock.

Perusal of the notes and discussion with parents will establish which children need to be immunized. Alternatively, a computer scheme may be programmed to produce a list of the immunization state of each school child.

Courses of diphtheria, tetanus and whooping cough may be completed at any time, however long the interval since commencement, and it is only necessary to re-start a polio course if the child was previously immunized with inactivated polio vaccine. Uptake of immunization is usually higher in areas which have a computer operated system and once the defaulter's name and address is pin-pointed by the system, consent forms and information may be sent to the parents. Uptake may be low because of either movement of families, manually operated recording and appointment systems, or the inability of parents to understand the literature produced by the computer. Under these circumstances the nurse and the doctor may wish to organize some health education sessions for the parents and teachers before running some sessions in the school.

Immunizations appropriate for school-age children, namely BCG, rubella and boosters of polio and tetanus, may be either combined with medical examinations or organized on an individual basis, depending on the preference of the doctor. The latter method is more common as this enables large numbers of children to be immunized and avoids extra administrative work.

BCG The incidence of tuberculosis in the population has declined considerably and because of the high cost of routine chest X-ray and BCG vaccination programmes, consideration may in the future be given to offering this to high risk groups only. Those who are most susceptible come from Pakistan, Bangladesh, India, Africa, West Indies and Ireland, although the likelihood of developing tuberculosis decreases the longer they live in this country.[3] At present it is important that all new entrant school children recently arrived from these countries should be offered BCG protection. Consent to this may present problems when parents do not speak English and are unable to read information in their native language. Arrangements may need to be made for an interpreter to explain the importance of immunization. Some areas are also offering BCG at birth or at school entry.

BCG should not be considered for children who have had a live vaccine less than three weeks ago, who are on immunosuppressive treatment, or who suffer from eczema or chronic skin complaints. A Mantoux or Heaf skin test is necessary to assess whether BCG should be offered, the latter being the more usual method as it is very quick and allows more children to be seen in a session. A small amount of BCG is placed on the left arm and the Heaf gun inflicts six small punctures. Two guns will be needed to allow for each to be passed through a spirit flame, between each child.

One week following, the skin tests are inspected for reactions as illustrated in Fig. 24. (*Negative* no reaction; faint signs of puncture marks. *Positive*, grade 1 reaction to at least four punctures; induration 1 mm in diameter around each puncture. *Grade 2* induration 2 mm in diameter around each puncture; slight oedema joining all or some areas of induration. *Grade 3* more intensive induration; more that 2 mm in diameter with oedema and induration between puncture marks forming a ring pattern. *Grade 4* complete disc of induration 5–10 mm in diameter. *Grade 4+* disc of induration more than 10 mm in diameter, may be ulceration in addition.) A very small or no reaction (*grade 1*) indicates that there is probably no immunity, and BCG should be offered. A moderate reaction (*grade 2*) indicates sufficient natural immunity and BCG is unnecessary. A severe reaction (*grades 3* and *4*) indicates that the child will need to be referred to the chest clinic for investigation.

BCG vaccination has become a lot easier since the introduction of the jet gun. However, the instructions for sterility should be carefully followed and arrangements may need to be made with the district central sterile supply department. A suggested sequence for immunization is as follows:

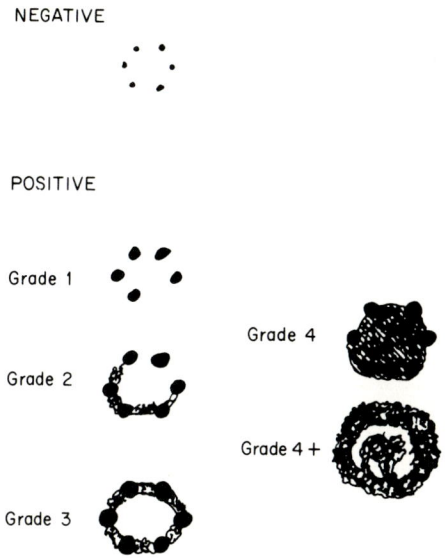

NEGATIVE

POSITIVE

Grade 1

Grade 2

Grade 3

Grade 4

Grade 4 +

Fig. 24. Heaf test reactions. (Fig. 4, p. 135 The Field Worker in Immigrant Health *edited by J. S. Dodge, Granada Publishing Ltd)*

a. Pre-school entry. Check immunization state when parents register with school and advise accordingly. Arrange for any consent forms to be signed.

b. Beginning of term. Check records of all children in the age group. (All will need a skin test, whether or not reported to have had BCG.)

c. 3 to 4 weeks before. Arrange health education, i.e. talks, posters, leaflets.

d. 2 to 3 weeks before. Arrange for all outstanding consents to be signed. Contact any parents who do not return forms and discuss.

The following skin test is required for BCG:

Skin test Children usually line up by class and file into the medical room. Left arm is skin-tested. Batch number is entered on the certificate and it is dated and signed.

1 week later Skin tests checked. BCG carried out as required and no further immunization should be given in that arm for three months. Severe reactions referred to chest clinic.

6 to 8 weeks BCG site inspected, reaction recorded. This includes the state of suppuration of scabs. Any swelling, swollen glands and severe reactions need to be reported to the doctor. Absence of reaction or large numbers of severe reactions might indicate a bad batch of vaccine or faulty technique. Suppurating wounds should be dressed with airstrip dressings. Water-proof dressing may be allowed for swimming but should be removed immediately afterwards. Adverse reactions are notified to the DHSS Adverse Reactions Sub-Committee on the Safety of Medicines.

Rubella A sequence similar to that for BCG testing may be used for rubella vaccination (except skin testing, which is not required). All girls whether reported to have had rubella or not should be offered the vaccine, unless there is any possible likelihood of pregnancy, otherwise the contraindications apply as for BCG. Rubella is often given six weeks following BCG so that the BCG site may be inspected at the same time (the minimum period allowed between BCG and rubella being three weeks).

Polio boosters These should be given before leaving school, unless the child had a reaction on the first occasion or has developed a hypersensitivity to penicillin, streptomycin or neomycin, or is suffering from a gastrointestinal disturbance.

Tetanus booster This should also be given before leaving school, unless a booster dose has recently been administered.

Identification

A sickening or infected child may be found in any of the following ways:

   a. by the teacher;
   b. during nurse's yearly health check or selective survey;
   c. a note from the parent or a doctor's certificate.

   a. Teachers need to be alert for the genuinely sick child and an experienced teacher or nurse will know which child really has a headache and which is a pre-maths class malingerer. A child who seems listless, inattentive, has puffy watery eyes, a cough or cold, and complains of feeling unwell, should be excused from class and allowed to lie down away from the other children but close to adult supervision. The parent should be contacted which may not be easy if the mother is working and the school has not kept up to date information as to her whereabouts. Other relatives may be contactable. Under no circumstances should a child be sent home to an empty house but kept in school until the mother arrives. Alternatively, the child could be accompanied home by an adult if there is a responsible person in the home. Should the child's condition deteriorate in the mother's absence, the head teacher acts in loco parentis, and the family practitioner should be called to advise.

   b. The nurse may discover children suffering from infectious diseases during her surveys (detailed in Chapter 9) or indeed they may come to light at medical examinations or during visits to the school.

   c. When a child is absent from school, the mother may inform the school by note or telephone, giving the reason, otherwise the education welfare officer will visit to discover why the child is absent and in the event of illness, will request a doctor's certificate. Sometimes this may be difficult to obtain as it is not always in the best interests of other patients to have infectious children brought to the surgery and the family practitioner may be hard pressed to visit the home. A charge for a certificate may deter single parents or poorer families from requesting one.

The head teacher usually sends a written return of absences through illness to the medical officer for environmental health and the area specialist in community medicine. If a number of children appear to be absent for similar reasons, for example sore throats or diarrhoea and cases of infectious diseases have been confirmed by family practitioners, the area specialist or the medical officer for environmental health may then ask that further investigations be made.

Contact Tracing and Action in School

The child suspected of suffering from infectious disease should be excluded from school until the diagnosis has been disproved by the family practitioner or the recommended exclusion period has passed. On confirmation of the diagnosis, the medical officer for environmental health may request that all contacts have nose and throat swabs for airborne infections, for example diphtheria or streptococcal respiratory infection, and specimens of faeces and rectal swabs for faecal-borne infections, for example bacillary dysentery, food poisoning, or typhoid. The school nurse or the environmental health officers may carry this out, depending on the type and size of the outbreak and the agreed local procedure. These specimens will be analysed by the public health laboratory service.

The whole school may be involved or only immediate contacts, and it is then necessary to establish accurately who these were. Contacts will be those infected from the original source and those secondarily infected from subsequent cases. Therefore, it is essential to understand the incubation period of the particular illness, i.e. the time between catching the infections and the development of signs and symptoms. Once this is known it can be established on which day the infection was caught and by following the actions of the ill child on that day, including the family and method of travel to the school, it will be possible to establish the source. This is very important in infections caught from carriers (those who do not develop the illness but carry the infection) or infected food.

With the help of the teachers, a list of all contacts should be made. They should be inspected for any symptoms, swabs taken as required by the doctor and immunization offered if appropriate. Children who have previously been immunized may be given a booster dose. The school staff, the parents and the nurse and doctor should not be forgotten as all investigations and protective measures apply equally to them as to the children. During an outbreak the nurse should visit the school daily, if possible, to check the class-rooms for any suspicious cases.

Contact Tracing and Action in the Home

Similarly, contacts in the home and the community will need to be traced and appropriate swabs and immunizations completed. These activities are usually jointly undertaken by the environmental health officers and members of the community nursing staff.

Home nursing With suitable nursing support, parents ought to be able to nurse children with chicken-pox, mumps or measles, at home. However, lone parents may be working and fear that they may lose their job through absence because of the child's illness. Consequently, the child may be left at home alone ill with little or no care or food during the day. Other parents find it difficult to understand what care is needed often because no one has taken the trouble to explain the nursing requirements. Indeed, many children are still admitted to the isolation hospitals for social reasons and not because they need isolation nursing. The school nurse ought to be sufficiently informed about the home to identify a child likely to find himself in such a plight. A home visit should then be made either by the district nurse, paediatric home care nurse or perhaps the school nurse, depending on local nursing policy. The principles of nursing care, diet and suitable occupational play material should be explained and demonstrated.

Isolation Nursing in Residential Units

When children are away from home, arrangements for suitable nursing need to be made in the school or hostel. Most residential establishments have a number of designated sick rooms although when large numbers of children develop infectious diseases, for example during an epidemic of influenza, there may not be a large enough number. Temporary arrangements will then have to be made to allocate certain rooms or dormitories for sick children to be nursed in. Pleasant rooms near to the toilets should be selected and healthy children should be transferred elsewhere. Children are less lonely when nursed together, particularly when barrier nursing is required. This should be carried out as follows:

1. Thorough handwashing following any handling of the child.
2. Immediate disposal by burning of all soiled dressings and tissues.
3. Frequent changes of clothing and sheets which should be laundered at high temperatures—suitable arrangements should be made with the laundry.
4. All feeding utensils should be sterilized in the dishwasher or kept and washed separately and rinsed with boiling water; alternatively, disposable items may be used.
5. Urine and faeces treated before disposal with disinfectant as recommended by the doctor, if necessary.
6. Room should be cleaned by damp dusting and mopping.

Arrangements need to be made for frequent fluids to be provided and small appetizing light meals. Children get very lonely, particularly if they are on their own, and the time seems very long as they get better. Suitable activities and amusements need to be organized and frequent visits made to the sick room to talk to the child. Ensure that there is communication with parents and school friends. Following recovery the room needs to be thoroughly cleaned and aired and all items disinfected or boiled, as appropriate.

Action on Return to School

The severity of infectious diseases varies as indeed will the diet and nursing care; consequently, some children may return to school feeling tired and listless. For a few days these children may need a little extra care and attention and encouragement to eat.

CONTAGIOUS DISEASES

There are a number of very contagious diseases which are not notifiable but are commonly found in school, and nurses have a major role to play in the care and control of these. They fall into the following four main groups:

1. Parasitic   pediculosis; scabies; worms.
2. Fungal   ringworm (tinea) of scalp, body, feet (athlete's foot), nails.
3. Viral   includes warts, i.e. both body and plantar warts (commonly known as varrucae); herpes.
4. Bacterial   these include boils, carbuncles, infected lacerations; impetigo; conjunctivitis.

The purpose of the nurse's hygiene rota is to discover these contagious diseases and prevent their spread throughout the school. She may see all the children routinely at the beginning of the school term, and subsequently as a result of referral from a parent or member of the school staff.

Her work will be reduced considerably if she understands thoroughly the method of spread and the value of good contact-tracing and health education. There is no use allowing an infected child to return to class and infect other children, or in inspecting all the children on one day and failing to clear absentees before their return to class. Treating a child in isolation without including the family and other members of the household is a waste of time and the disease is highly likely to be recurrent: the child may either have infected other members of the family or the family may be the source of infection for the child, and hence it becomes a vicious circle. Therefore, it is essential that everyone in the house is treated and if it is likely that any instructions will not be carried out, a home visit must be made to see that they are. Contacts include all members of the family living in the home and any regular visitors or close contacts they may have. School pets should also be inspected as occasionally they may be a source of infection. Should this be the case the environmental health officer should be informed and measures will be taken to dispose of the animal.

Once treatment has been commenced, children can usually return to school except in cases of ringworm of the scalp which is difficult to cover and can be unsightly and embarrassing for the child. Problems may arise, however, with short time medication such as antibiotics which may need to be given during the day. Where possible, doctors need to prescribe drugs which can be taken out of school hours or, alternatively, arrangements may be made in the school with the head teacher and the school nurse. General principles outlined on p. 110 apply.

Parasitic Infections

Pediculosis Pediculosis of infection with lice can be of the head (capitas), body (corporis) or pubic parts (pubis). Head infestation is by far the most usual type seen by the school nurse although body and pubic lice may be more common than we think. Some parents get very agitated about head lice, believing wrongly that they occur only in dirty children and that, therefore, a slight is cast on their care of the child. Lice are easily transferred when children's heads are in close contact and short hair, contrary to popular belief, may make the process even easier.

The lice live close to the head and the nits (eggs) usually take between 6 and 16 days to hatch, depending on the temperature (Fig. 25). Following hatching the empty shell remains cemented to the hair until it is cut off, usually by using a special fine comb with a sharp blade which cuts the hair just removing the nit. Diagnosis is described on p. 127. The present recommended treatment is lotion containing malathion or carboryl, rubbed into the dry hair and left for 24 hours before shampooing with an ordinary shampoo. Shampoos containing insecticide are not recommended as the detergent in the shampoo inhibits the action of the insecticide on the lice. Outbreaks tend to be more common following school holidays, particularly in September.

Nursing action All the children in the school should be examined on the same day and any children absent should be examined before being allowed back to class. This avoids infected children re-infecting those already seen. Teams of nurses or auxiliaries may work together to achieve this in large schools.

1. Issue lotion and instructions for cleansing to the parents of infected children. The whole family should be treated. Alternatively, they may attend the local authority cleansing centre.
2. Inspect the child's hair on the following morning before the child enters school. If several children need to be seen, time can be saved by smelling the hair to confirm treatment rather than re-examining it.
3. Any child still infested should be excluded by the head teacher.

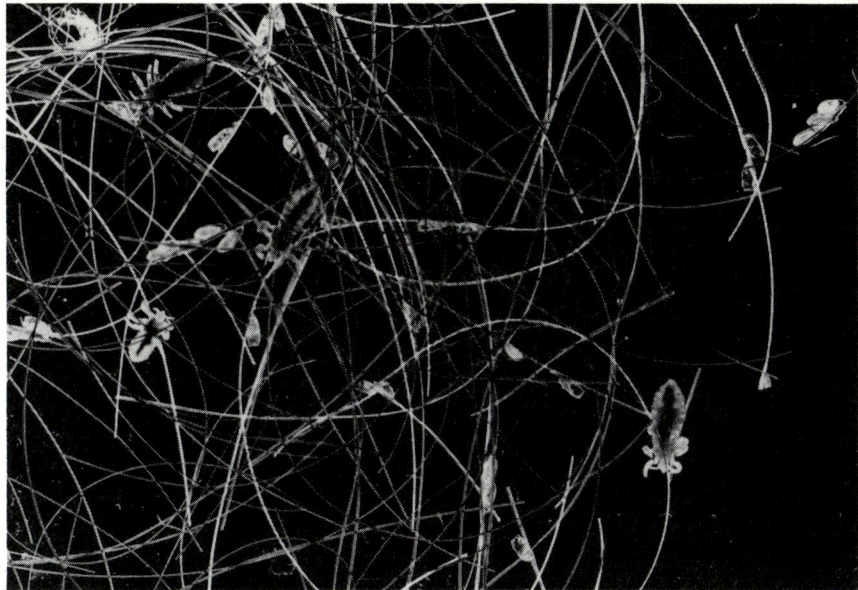

Fig. 25. Nits and lice in the hair. (James Webb)

Under the 1944 Education Act, Section 54 (i) to (viii), any authorized officer of the education authority may serve a notice on the parent of a pupil requiring the pupil to be treated. If this is not carried out within a specified time, which must not be less than 24 hours, the child may be removed to the cleansing station and treated accordingly.

If following treatment the pupil is again found to be verminous, the education authority may, if they can prove this is due to neglect on the part of the parent, take the parents to court where they may be liable to a fine.

Scabies This is caused by a small mite burrowing and reproducing beneath the skin. Usually it presents in reddish lines, between the fingers and on the wrists or back of the hand and sometimes it is seen on the trunk (Fig. 26). It causes itching, particularly when the body is warm and it is also very contagious. Contaminated bed-clothes, towels and clothing are a source of infection.

The present treatment is for the infected child to be given a hot bath and all the burrow lines of the mite should be thoroughly scrubbed with a nail brush (see Fig. 26). The body should not be dried but painted all over from the neck downwards with 25% emulsion of benzl benzoate. A second coat is applied as soon as the first is dry. After 24 hours repeat the two applications of the lotion only. On the third day the child has a bath and a set of clean clothes.

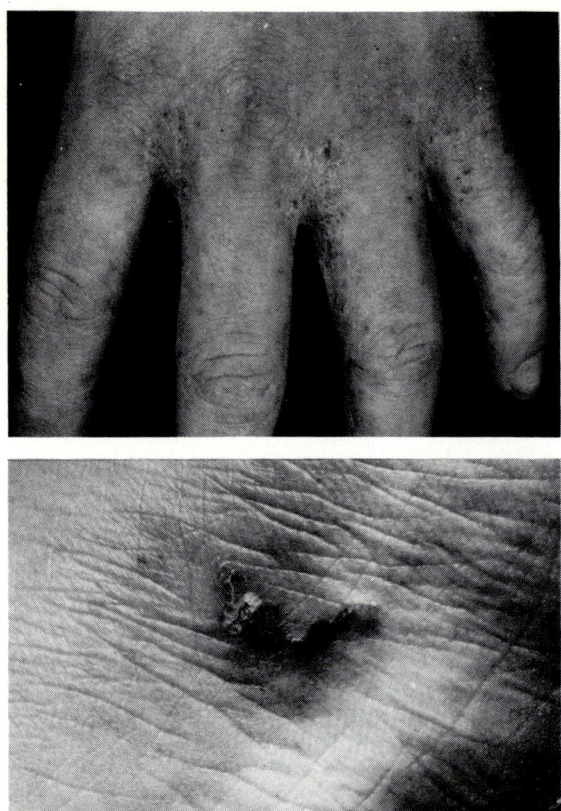

Fig. 26. Top: *Typical distribution of scabies between fingers.* Bottom: *Typical burrow line of the mite.* (*Figs 26, 27, 28: Institute of Dermatology*)

Nursing action
1. Contact the mother and arrange for child to be seen by the family practitioner or attend the bathing centre.
2. Examine all other children who are likely to have had contact and arrange treatment for them also.
3. Home visit to trace contacts and advise them to see the general practitioner or attend the bathing centre.
4. Advise mother to boil all clothing or iron with a hot iron. Arrange any auto-cleansing of bed-clothes with the environmental health department. Any items difficult to cleanse should be left unused for three weeks when the parasites will have died.
5. Child may return to school following treatment.

Worms The most common types found in children are thread worms (oxyuriasis) which show up in the stools as small white threads. Usually ingested from infected food or fingers. The child usually complains of sleeplessness, itching around the anus and is generally irritable. Round worms (ascaris lumbricadies) though less common, may also be found particularly in children who have immigrated or returned from holidays in tropical countries. The child may complain of abdominal pains, diarrhoea or vomiting. They are usually contracted via the feet while walking barefoot on infested ground or through taking infected food or water. Diagnosis is by examination of the stool to find the worms which range from about 12 to 30 cm in length. The doctor may prescribe pripsen or vanguin for thread worms and piperazine citrate and a saline purge 24 hours later for round worms.

Nursing action
1. See that attention is paid to hygiene, particularly washing of hands and finger nails. There should be satisfactory sanitary arrangements to dispose of faeces and no child with round worms should be allowed to defecate on the ground.
2. Frequent changes of bed linen and night clothes. Child should sleep alone.

Other worms which need mention as they are particularly dangerous to young children are *Toxocara canis* and *Cati*. These are found in cats and dogs which have not been dewormed. The eggs are passed in the excreta which if handled by a child causes toxocariasis. It can also cause blindness and damage to the heart and lungs. Consequently, it is extremely important to see that playgrounds and sand pits are free from animal excreta. Pets should be dewormed frequently and the faeces properly disposed of and children be discouraged from handling strange dogs and cats.

Fungal Infections

Ringworm Ringworm may occur on the scalp (*Tinea capitis*), body (*Tinea corporis*), feet (*Tinea pedis*, or athlete's foot), or nails (*Tinea unguium*). They may be contracted from animals, particularly dogs and possibly from contaminated showers, floors and benches, usually in gyms and swimming baths.

Tinea capitis may be confused with patches of alopecia seen particularly in West Indian and African children when the hair has been tightly plaited. Certain diagnosis can only be made by using a Wood's Lamp.

Nursing action
1. Ask the parents to take the child to the family practitioner to confirm diagnosis and prescribe treatment.
2. Home visit to advise any contacts to seek treatment. Affected pets should be treated by the veterinary surgeon.
3. Advise mother to boil or wash in very hot water any socks, woolly hats and gloves.

4. Arrange autocleansing for any school clothing used for theatrical performances or dressing-up likely to have been infected.
5. Child should return to school as soon as treatment is commenced and lesions are covered.

Viral Infections

Warts or varrucae These are caused by a virus infection entering a lesion or skin puncture. They may be seen on the hands, fingers or nails (varrucae vulgaris) or on the face and knees (varrucae plana), or on the feet (varrucae planteris or plantar warts) (see Fig. 27). The incubation period may be one to six months and the infection seems to be particularly easy to catch around swimming pools. Little is known about the virus and some people seem to be immune and some very susceptible, particularly if taking steroids or immunosuppressive drugs. It is thought that most warts heal spontaneously and disappear within 3 to 5 years. Treatment is probably only necessary if they are painful, inhibiting

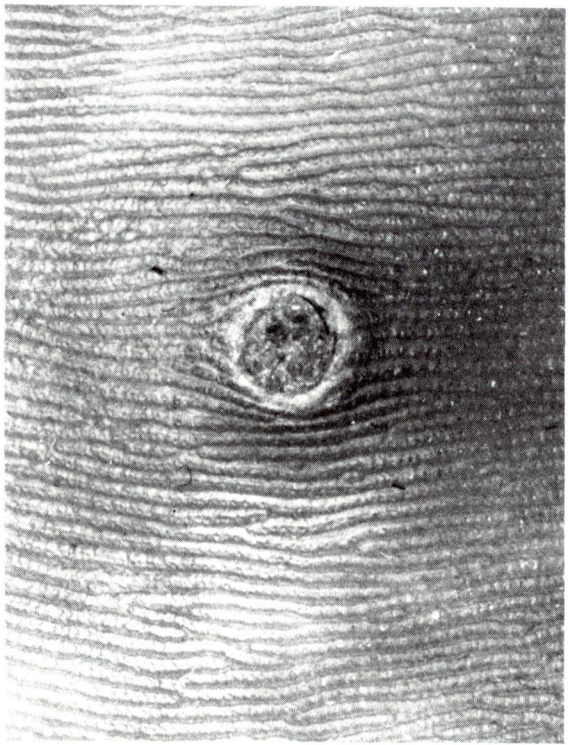

Fig. 27. Typical varrucae on the sole of the right foot.

activities or to prevent spreading to other children. Treatment is generally by strapping a pad soaked in formaldehyde solution to the varrucae nightly, soaking in hot water, followed by chaffing with pumice-stone or sandpaper. Persistent painful warts may be removed by applying carbon dioxide snow or liquid nitrogen to freeze them out; alternatively, cautery or diathermy will burn them.

Nursing Action
1. Refer to family practitioner, varrucae or dermatology clinic according to local procedure, for confirmation of diagnosis and treatment.
2. Reassure parents and teaching staff and suggest that swimming pool surrounds and showers are mopped frequently and kept as dry as possible. Socks or ballet shoes could be worn for gymnastics although children are less likely to catch infection on dry clean floors. Plastasox could be advised for swimming.

Herpes simplex This often appears following colds or 'flu and is usually seen on the lips or the edges of the nose. Inflammation is generally followed by vesicles and yellow crusts and it has a tendency to occur in the same spot. It usually resolves itself after a few days but persistent serious cases should be referred to the doctor for treatment.

Nursing Action
1. Advise on general hygiene.
2. Ensure that towels and face flannels are not used by other children or members of the family.

Bacterial Infections

The most common of these is *Staphylococcus aureus*. Infected hair follicles may result in boils or carbuncles, often seen around the neck and base of the hair. They usually respond to treatment with topical antibiotics.

Impetigo (see Fig. 28) is distinguished by the golden crusted lesions usually seen on the face, particularly around the nose, ears and scalp. It spreads easily and is frequently the result of scratching and irritation caused by parasitic infestation.

Nursing Action
1. Examine for parasitic infection and if confirmed follow the procedure and treat as already described.
2. Arrange for doctor to prescribe antibiotic treatment for impetigo.
3. Child should be excluded from school until recovered.

Conjunctivitis Infective conjunctivitis usually presents with yellow mucus discharge and the eyelids are usually stuck together following sleep. The cause is most likely to be bacterial or fungal infection.

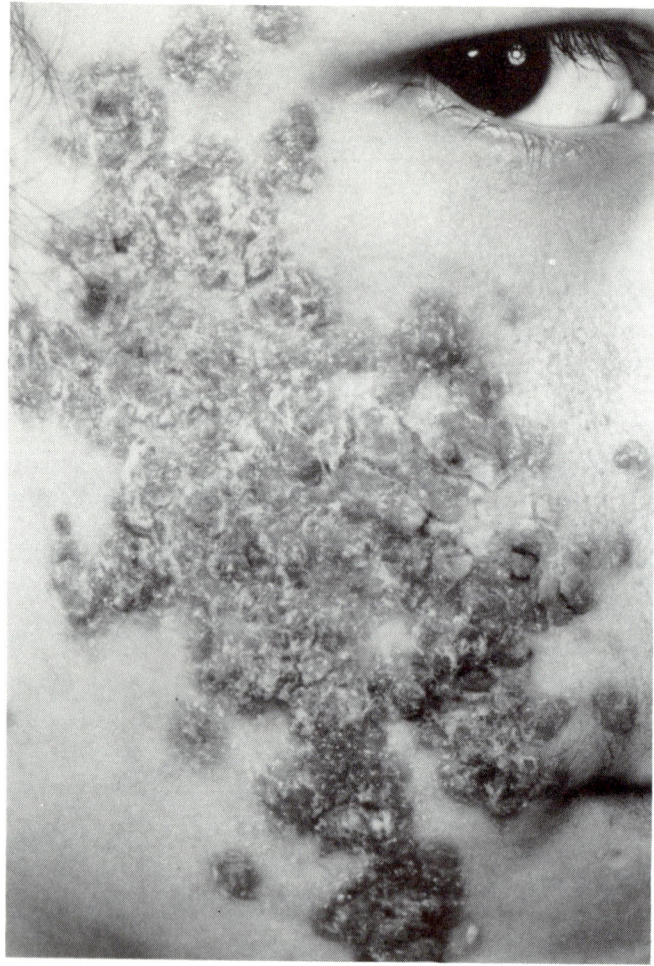

Fig. 28. Impetigo.

Nursing action
1. Refer to doctor for diagnosis and treatment.
2. Advise family on general hygiene. Particularly important that face-flannels and towels are not used by others.

REFERENCES

1. Turtle, de Bec (1975) *Handbook of School Health Officers of Schools Association.* London: H. K. Lewis.

2. DHSS & DES (1977) *Memorandum on the Control of Infectious Diseases in School.* London: HMSO.
3. Br. Thoracic & Tuberculosis Association. (1975) Tuberculosis among immigrants—related to length of residence in England and Wales. *Br. med. J.,* 3, pp. 698–699.

FURTHER READING

Editorial (1972) Plantar Warts. *Br. med.J.,* **ii**, p. 723.
DHSS (1972) *Immunization Against Infectious Diseases.* London: HMSO.
DHSS (1977) *Memorandum on the Control of Infectious Diseases in School.* London: HMSO.
DHSS CM01/74 (1974) *Vaccination Procedures.* London: HMSO.
Dubay, E. C. & Grubb, R. D. (1973) *Infection Prevention and Control.* St Louis, U.S.A.: C. V. Mosby.
Johnston, D. F. (1968) *Essentials of Communicable Disease with Nursing Principles,* 5th ed. London: Faber & Faber.
Slack, P. A. (1976) Head infestation. *Nursing Times,* **72**, 6, pp. 225–227.

CHILDREN'S BOOKS

Cass, J. (1976) *Milly Mouses Measles.* London: Kaye & Ward. A picture book describing how the mice go for measles immunization. 3 + years.
Wolde, G. (1975) *Emma and the Measles.* Leicester: Brockhampton.

Discussion Topics

1. A number of children are absent with infectious diseases. What reasons might necessitate home visits and by whom?

2. A child with an infected laceration has been prescribed antibiotics by the family practitioner. He arrives in school with some drugs wrapped in a paper handkerchief and hands them to the teacher. The head teacher refuses to handle or give the drugs and says the child must stay at home until he is better. Both parents are out working. How might the situation be solved?

3. Three children recently arrived from Pakistan are admitted to the school.

Would this require you to take any action and would you anticipate any problems?

4. You attend a school function and find yourself with a group of mothers who are discussing their children's many coughs and colds. The local doctor is not keen to prescribe antibiotics and they are very critical of him. What might you tell them about immunological development.

5. You are passing the school playground in the evening and you notice several stray animals inside and the sand pit in particular is badly fouled. How would you deal with the situation?

6. There is a very low uptake of BCG and rubella vaccination in the school. Consider any reasons for this and suggest ways in which you might increase acceptance.

11
Health Education

The purpose of health education is quite simply to persuade people to adopt health practices which will prevent their mind or body from becoming ill. Successful health education could have enormous implications not only for the individual but for our country and the world in general. A few simple examples are:

1. If people drove and cycled more safely and were careful crossing roads, the number of road accidents would be reduced and the demand on hospital beds and medical care for road casualties would be drastically reduced, thus releasing money for other projects. The cost of road accidents in 1976 was estimated to be in the region of £415 million.[1]
2. If more children developed a keen interest in physical pursuits which they carried on into adult life, it is likely that this would have a significant effect on the incidence of coronary artery disease, thereby reducing the number of lonely, depressed and dependent widows in the 60-year-old age group.
3. If most mothers breast-fed their babies the likelihood of developing obesity, allergies and possibly arterial disease[2] from artificial milk would decrease. This would reduce individual discomfort and misery and the demand on medical services, not to mention school nurse work-load.
4. If more children during their school life developed keen interests in the subjects taught or in completing the tasks set, the way would be paved for enjoying one's job and recreation, and providing a means to making friends and sharing interests, thereby reducing discontent and loneliness. The number of days lost to industry through sickness would be reduced as well as the demands on family practitioner, psychiatric and social work services.

From these examples it can be seen that although the aim is simple the subject is complex, interwoven with the total aim of education and thus covering the entire school curricula and highlighting deficiencies or absences from it. Giving information is not sufficient in itself as there is no guarantee that the child will be interested enough to absorb it or more importantly, having acquired the information will act upon it.

The school health team's responsibilities towards health teaching include:

1. Helping to identify the health needs of the children and their community.
2. Acting as a professional link for teachers giving them advice on current medical research and thinking.
3. Assisting by answering questions and participating in specialist topics.
4. Using their knowledge of local resources to assist in programme planning (recruiting other specialists or indicating possible fields for project work).
5. Influencing the general health practice and organization within the school by advice and example.
6. Providing individual health teaching and counselling to children on a one-to-one basis as necessary or as requested by the child, the parents or the teaching staff.

Teaching is the responsibility of teachers and only qualified teachers should be engaged in this, other than on a specialist topic on which a nurse or doctor may be invited to speak or answer questions. The teachers involved in curricula planning should ensure that the school health team are represented or consulted on their plans so that the children are not given conflicting information and that questions subsequently presented to the health staff and arising from the teaching may be anticipated and dealt with more satisfactorily. It also presents an opportunity to consider some of the effects of aspects of the programme on children who may be attending specialist clinics or receiving services likely to be discussed.

To plan a health education programme, the following questions need to be asked.

Who Teaches Health Education?

Various aspects of health education can be demonstrated through a variety of subjects—practical and physical information through biology, science and home economics; social, historical and organizational aspects through English, history and geography; and the emotional and moral questions of human relationships through literature, pastoral tutorial groups, religious education and drama. Schools vary as to who takes overall responsibility. Some schools have appointed health education co-ordinators or the responsibility has been added to an existing post such as head of biology, house tutor or religious education teacher. Sometimes a school may even have a health education committee consisting of interested members of the staff and even representatives of the parents and the children. However, there are many schools, particularly boys' schools, which have no arrangements for health education although various education reports, including the 1944 Education Act, the Plowden Report and more recently the Court Report, have stressed the value of educating for health as an important preparation for adult life. The head teacher should be asked to explain the arrangements within the school and can see that the school health team are given the facility to contribute appropriately.

When a nurse is asked to contribute by actually teaching or holding a discussion group, she should ensure that she is adequately informed about what exactly is required and in what context: Is this part of a planned continuous programme? What ages are the children and how much will they understand? Have the children had any previous information on the topic? How many will there be and where will it take place? Is there a possibility of using audio-visual aids and how is this arranged? Will there be further follow-up?

The nurse who has not previously participated in a teaching programme should explain that to the teacher and seek guidance on preparation and presentation. There is no reason why she should not ask to sit in as an observer in the class on one or two occasions. This type of information and preparation is necessary for success and avoids the sort of disastrous situations where the inexperienced nurse is faced with an assembly hall of 200 children of mixed age groups and abilities and is required to talk about sex. A nurse who feels unable to contribute to teaching a group or class should say so and see that some other nurse or health visitor is found to do this. Alternatively, she can see that the teacher is given sufficient information to undertake the teaching while the nurse sits in and contributes to questions and discussion. Teaching in a one to one situation should take place at any time when questions are asked or the opportunity arises.

The possible contribution of external help should not be forgotten. Many schools ask members of the community, such as the police or road safety officers, to participate in their programme. Other possibilities include a representative from the local authority housing department, particularly where large numbers of children come from families who have not succeeded in managing their housing arrangements satisfactorily. Young parents and babies may usefully contribute to a child development or parenthood programme (see Fig. 29).

The children may be encouraged to contribute or take part in activities outside the school which add to the health teaching. The education youth service can encourage involvement in activities such as the St John Ambulance Brigade or the Red Cross. The school children might be encouraged to participate as volunteers in the local children's ward reading and playing with younger children, putting on an entertainment or repairing broken toys in the school workshop.

The local children's library encourages children to read, and organizes story-telling sessions as well as activities for parents during school holidays. Health teaching may also be included and relevant novels or practical work books stocked and recommended, or read to the children (see Fig. 30). The children's librarian may also be extremely helpful in suggesting further suitable books on

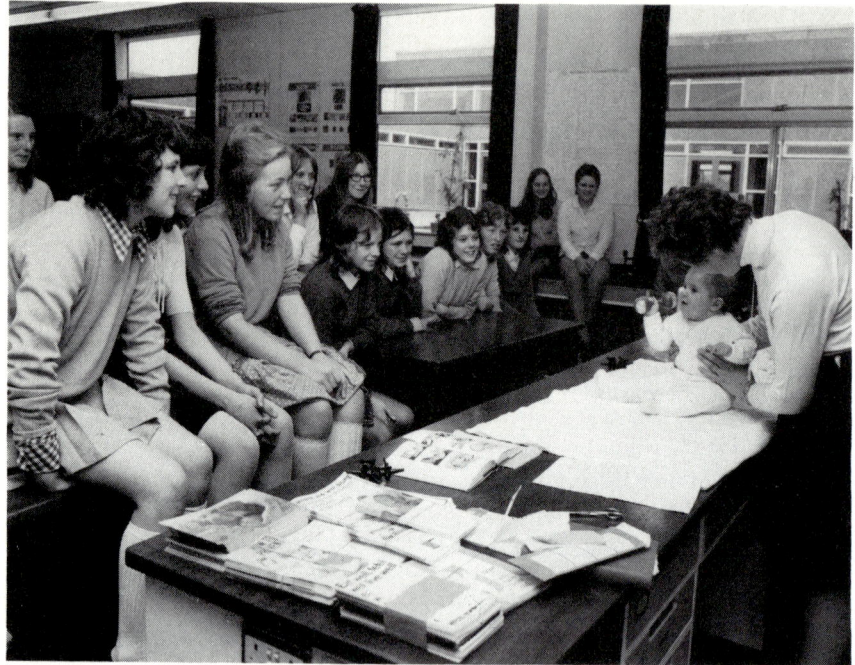

Fig. 29. Demonstrating practical child development. (Central Office of Information)

health topics, besides those listed in this book, which might be included in the school library or used by the nurse to complement individual health teaching during or in preparation for health checks, medical examinations or immunization sessions.

What Needs to be Taught?

Adults may have varying ideas about what needs to be taught. However, the ultimate choice should be related to the prevalence of health needs: firstly in the school community; secondly, in the local area; and thirdly, the country as a whole. Some of these will be specific to individual schools and some will be common locally or nationally, and teaching planned within the school can supplement or take advantage of local or national campaigns. The use of seat-belts and anti-smoking propaganda are typical examples. The school health team should know what the particular health problems of the school are, both from taking note of their own medical and social records, statistical returns, or keeping account of suspected difficulties.

Fig. 30. Selection of children's books concerning various aspects of health.

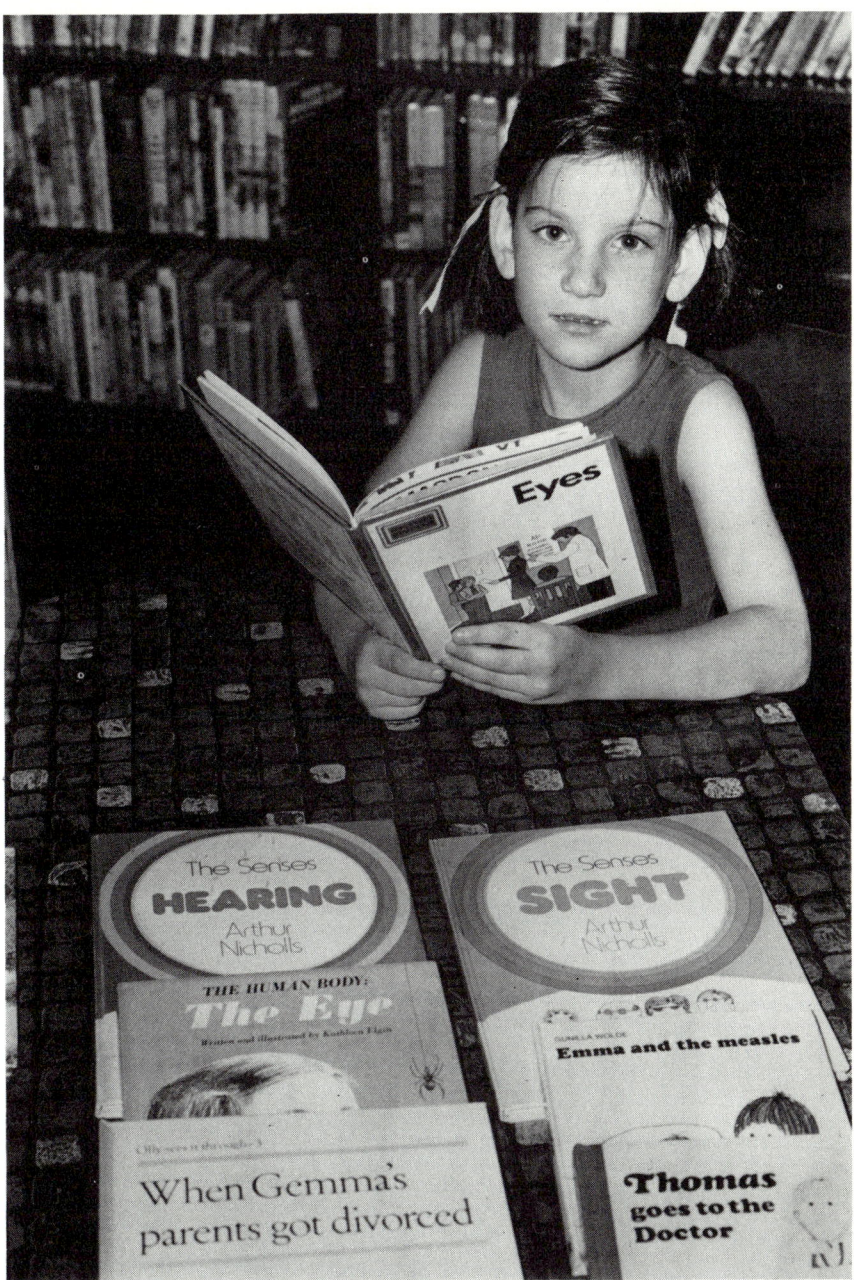

A picture might emerge as follows: *Physical*—malnutrition (obesity or rickets); dental caries; poor personal hygiene; frequent absences arising from dysmenorrhoea; several children injured in road accidents. *Social*—poor housing; poor parental house-keeping and financial management of the home; poor parental care; parental divorce. *Emotional*—truancy; promiscuity; school-girl pregnancies; adolescent petty theft and violence. *Organization*—failed appointments for medical examinations; large number of refusals for BCG.

It is obvious from such a picture that many of the problems are interrelated. The emotional difficulties probably stem from the social circumstances; indeed, the physical problems may also arise from them.

School health education also has a secondary effect in that parents may be influenced either directly through discussion at parent–teacher associations or indirectly through the teaching the children have received. An example might be seen among immigrant children who have been poorly nourished because their parents are unable to afford their native foods and do not know how to use cheaper British substitutes to achieve the same result. The domestic science teacher may become aware of the problem and plan her classes so that the girls learn how to cook their traditional dishes using English ingredients. This subsequently may influence the shopping habits of the parents.

We have, however, to decide what the broad *aims* of the programme will be, taking into consideration what is possible within the time available, the staff's capabilities and the specialist help available to be recruited from the community. Three aims emerging from the above list might be: to reduce the number of children injured by road accidents; to reduce dental caries; and to raise the standard of parenting in the next generation.

Having decided on the aims, it is then necessary to decide on the objectives of the programme. In other words, what is it that the children will do at the end of the teaching which will mean that the number of road accidents and dental caries are reduced and ensure that the next generation will prove better parents. Here the school health team can contribute by interpreting and advising the thinking of the medical and dental professions on these topics. This can be expanded for the teachers by supplying them with references or resource information on the reasons or research behind this thinking. Detailed objectives are not easy to set. However, we are a lot more certain as to the action required to reduce dental caries and road accidents than to improve parenting. Three of the main objectives which might be set to achieve the aims could be:

1. Children will only cross roads when it is safe to do so.
2. Children will no longer eat sweet snacks between meals.
3. When the child becomes a parent he or she will do the following:
    a. spend more time talking to the child,
    b. will play with the child,
    c. will understand how to prepare young children adquately for unavoid-able separation (illness of parent, admission of child to hospital).

Having decided on the objectives, the methods of teaching may be considered.

How Do We Teach It?

There are a wide variety of methods of group teaching which qualified teachers have learned to practice with varying degrees of skill. For this reason the methods to use for teaching are best left to them. However, it is important to understand something of the associated influences which affect the message whether it is put over in a one to one situation or a group.

Attitudes to the topics in question have a major influence on the timing and effectiveness of the teaching and it must always be remembered that we are trying to ensure that the information given will be put to practical daily use. This involves influencing attitudes during a time when they are being formed or much more difficult, changing attitudes already hardened (see Fig. 31). There is increasing evidence from surveys of attitudes[3] among young children on sex,

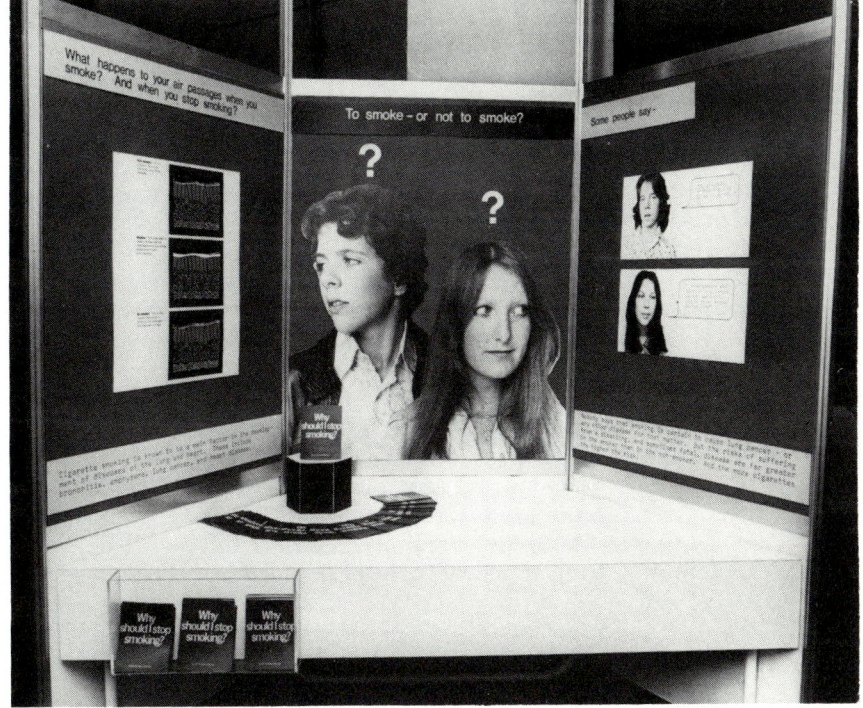

Fig. 31. The influences that form attitudes and their effect on accepting information. Boy: My grandad smoked and he lived to be 95. Girl: I knew someone who died of lung cancer at the age of 50 and he never smoked in his life. (The Health Education Council)

alcohol and smoking that concepts of these are already forming during the early primary years. Therefore, this is a time when success is most likely to be achieved. Starting in the secondary years is probably far too late and therefore programmes designed for teenagers should be a continuation of work started with the young school child.

There are, of course, teenagers and indeed parents who can be helped and influenced by a good school programme. This may involve the more difficult task of changing attitudes rather than influencing their formation, in which case it must be kept in mind that change is unlikely to happen unless the individual sees it as a means to an end and feels it to be of crucial personal importance. It is therefore essential to know what are seen as immediate goals and to demonstrate that the practice you are advocating will help individuals to achieve those goals. For example, the adolescents pictured in Fig. 31 may want to do well in sport; consequently, they will probably be able to see the disadvantages of smoking, if this aspect is presented to them. It is also important that the personal example and organizational practice of the school support rather than contradict the teaching.

Personal example This is extremely important in influencing children who learn from mimicking and emulating the practice of adults closest to them and admired by them. The parents have the most important early influence and later the school, to a considerable degree. Teachers and school staff who are considerate, clean and well-groomed, have good table manners and are sensitive to the children's needs, are careful to see that there is time for hand-washing before meals and after using the toilet, will have a far greater influence on the children's personal hygiene than hours of teaching about infections. The public are influenced by nursing examples which is why so many advertisements for patent medicines use a nursing image. A nurse who is admired and liked by the children and is careful about her own health can influence the children and other staff considerably. A nurse seen eating snacks between meals, not observing the rules of the road or not bothering to talk constructively to the children is hardly likely to encourage the objectives just outlined. Pop and sports stars also influence the children and can be shown as good examples. We have seen this used on television; for example, Jimmy Saville promoting seat-belts for safe driving. Personal experience of a practice is also important. A child or adolescent for whom the school health service has been helpful and beneficial will be more likely to see the value of occupational health, antenatal care, maternity and child health and screening services when they become adults.

School organization This is very important in encouraging the formation of good habits. If we examine our own daily life pattern it is easy to see that the time we spend cleaning our teeth, washing our hands after visiting the toilet, manner and time spent on eating food, type of food we enjoy, and other automatic actions and responses are habits that stretch far back into childhood and were learnt at home or in school. A good school recognizes this in its daily routine and allows sufficient time for these actions to be carried out satisfactorily (see Fig. 32). Where this is not happening attention should be drawn to the matter.

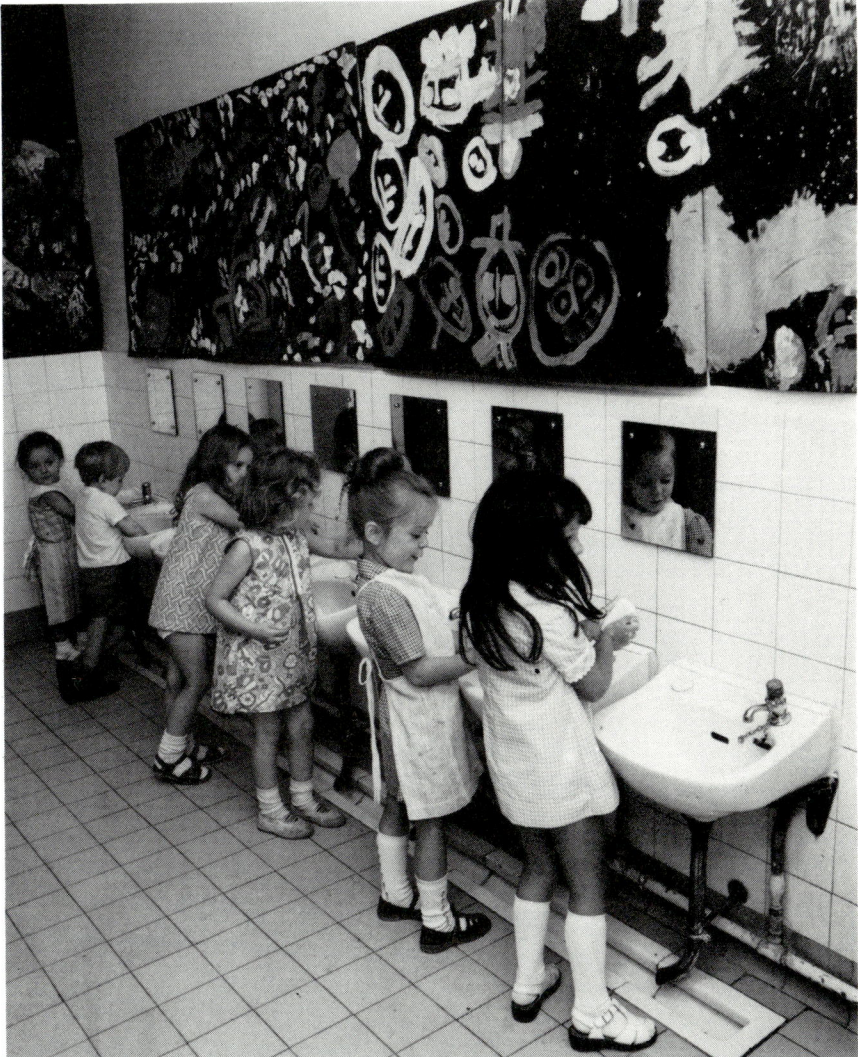

Fig. 32. Learning the habit of handwashing before meals in the nursery school. (Central Office of Information)

It is no good teaching about the digestive system if meals are wolfed in a couple of minutes or about nourishing tasty food if the school dinners are stodgy and uninteresting. Teaching children not to eat sweet snacks between meals so that their teeth may be preserved is totally undermined if the school continues to sell sweets or allows them to be brought to school.

Attention also needs to be given to the practical possibilities of continuing with certain interests into adult life such as sports. Some activities which are likely to be carried on to the end of life and shared between the sexes should be encouraged, walking and swimming being good examples.

Evaluation Any teaching should be assessed to see whether it was effective or not, and this should be a built-in part of the programme. At the beginning of the programme we defined what the child would be expected to do at the end of the teaching so we must test whether this has been achieved or not. This is important as otherwise our teaching may even have an adverse effect. This is easier than it sounds and is a field which is being studied by educationalists and psychologists alike. Examinations such as 'A' and 'O' levels test the amount of information a child has absorbed but it cannot test to what end the child will use that information. Skills may be tested as in the driving test but it is not possible to accurately examine, as yet, whether the application of the skill will always be applied in a way that pays due consideration to the safety of others. Teaching about drugs and sex has often been said to have had adverse effects, and we have little concrete proof either way. The NHS and the education service have important research fields to explore together as it is only when they can undertake long-term investigations into the effects of health teaching that we shall really understand the degree of benefit; for example, parentcraft teaching in school can only be evaluated when those children become parents themselves.

REFERENCES

1. DHSS (1976) *Prevention and Health—Everybody's Business*. London: HMSO.
2. Richards, M. P. M. (1974) *The Pros and Cons of Breast-feeding*. Unpublished available from unit for Research on the Medical Applications of Psychology, 5 Salisbury Villas, Station Road, Cambridge.
3. Schools Council Working Paper 57 (1976) *Health Education in Secondary Schools*. London: Evans/Methuen.

FURTHER READING

Dalzell-Ward, A. J. (1975) *Textbook of Health Education*. London: Tavistock.
DES (1973) *The Family in Society—Dimensions of Parenthood*, London: HMSO.
DES (1973) *The Family in Society—Preparation for Parenthood*, London: HMSO.
DES (1968) *Handbook of Health Education*. London: HMSO.
DES (1966) *Health in Education*. London: HMSO.
DES (1977) *Health Education in Schools*. London: HMSO.
Runswick, H. (1976) *Health Education—Practical Teaching Techniques*. Aylesbury, Buckinghamshire: HM & M.

USEFUL ADDRESSES AND INFORMATION

The Health Education Council
78 New Oxford Street
London WC1A 1AH.
Tel: 01 637 1881.

Nationally-funded body. They provide information and advice together with free teaching resource lists on a number of topics. Issue a *Health Education Bulletin* once every term to all schools, distributed by the local education authority. *The Health Education Council Project Materials* is due to be published in 1978 by Cambridge University Press.

The Schools Council
Information Section
160 Great Portland Street
London W1N 6LL.
Tel: 01 580 0352.

Issue a full list of all their working papers and curriculum bulletins. A working party set up in 1970 on Health Education resulted in the production of a series of projects and publications designed to help teachers and now being widely used.

School Radio and TV Broadcasts
The Secretary
School Broadcasting Council (30/BC)
BBC
London W1A 1AA.
Tel: 01 580 4468.

Programmes specifically for teachers to use in class frequently cover health, social and environmental topics. Advance information. Programmes usually available in most schools, otherwise may be obtained from the BBC.

Discussion Topics

1. A new teacher approaches you, telling you that she wants to start some health education teaching and would like your assistance. In what ways could you help her?

2. You are employed in a school where there is said to be no 'health education'. The teachers are uninterested and see health as a low priority. Consider ways in which you might seek to change their attitudes.

3. The school playground is always full of litter and some of the children have had minor accidents with broken glass and empty metal cans. Consider ways in which the school system might be used to alter this situation and the long-term attitudes of the staff and children.

4. You are employed in a school where much of your time is taken up with duties such as routine selective surveys for contagious diseases, home visits to follow-up failed appointments and parental non-attendance at medical examinations. Consider ways in which health education might be used to reduce this work-load. How might the time saved be allocated more beneficially?

5. One of the teachers says, 'Will you come and talk to my class about sex on Thursday next, please'. What is your reply?

6. Consider suitable health education materials which you might use in the medical room. How would you obtain them and in what ways might you use them?

12
Occupational Health and First-aid

Acquiring an education is a full-time occupation for 5 to 16-year-olds and is fraught with just as many hazards as many working situations. The risks of fire, accidents from gas and electricity, injuries from equipment in practical work departments and from chemicals and inflammable liquids in laboratories are just as likely to occur in schools as elsewhere. Indeed, the inexperience of the learning school child probably presents a greater risk.

The 1974 Health and Safety at Work Act was the first piece of comprehensive safety legislation to cover all sections of the population, including employees in educational establishments. The body appointed to see that the Act is enforced are the Health and Safety Executive who are represented by the Factory Inspectorate (see Environmental health p. 24). They have powers to take samples and investigate any premises where they feel there is cause for concern for the safety of the employees. The education authority has a responsibility for the safety of all staff employed in the school, together with visitors who include visiting staff such as the school nurse and also the pupils. The authority can in fact be prosecuted by the Health and Safety Executive and this has indeed happened. Consequently, education authorities are becoming more concerned. Investigations into all accidents in schools are starting to be set up and it is possible that within the next few years considerable change will take place in this field.

Occupational health in schools has declined in recent years, although ideally the responsibility for it should be met by the school health service. The school health services in independent schools have maintained their responsibility for general school health and safety but, unfortunately, this is not so in the majority of maintained schools.

Indeed, the following incidents reported by Mrs Allen of the Hampshire

School Matrons' Association illustrate the kind of accident which can occur and the need for adequate first-aid procedure together with thorough investigations to avoid reoccurrence.

1. David, aged 12 years David was being chased in the playground during the lunchtime break when he fell down some steps. The accident was reported to me verbally by another pupil, and members of the staff brought David into the medical room on a stretcher. He had sustained a Pott's fracture of the left ankle.

He was placed on the bed in the medical room with the left foot and leg slightly elevated on a pillow; David was in a slight stage of shock and in some degree of pain, and because of his age needed a lot of reassurance.

The ambulance was sent for as this was a case needing direct transport to hospital. I contacted his mother by 'phoning her at work, and her arrival at the school was a great source of comfort to David. The ambulance arrived and David's ankle was immobilized in a plastic inflatable splint. He was carefully lifted onto a stretcher and transported to the district hospital accompanied by his mother.

There his ankle was X-rayed and later he was taken to theatre where the fracture was reduced and the foot put into plaster. His fracture healed well and after two weeks he returned to school having suffered no ill effects. He is now able to take part in a full and active school life.

David was wearing rather high wedge shoes at the time of his accident, which might have attributed to it. This aspect of the incident was subsequently included in the school health education programme.

2. Christopher, aged 13 years Christopher was in a woodwork lesson when his work jammed between the table and the sanding disc; this dragged his left hand into the disc.

Christopher was being supervised at the time of the accident by the teacher in charge. He had been instructed in the correct use of the machine and was permitted to use it but not to hold the work at an angle to the table: this is what led directly to the accident. The accident was reported verbally by the teacher who accompanied Christopher to the medical room.

Christopher had sustained severe lacerations of his index and second fingers of his left hand. His hand was wrapped in a dressing and elevated in a sling and he was then transported to the local health centre which is some half a mile away. Here he was taken to the treatment room, laid on a couch and his hand cleaned whilst awaiting the arrival of the doctor. I tried to contact his mother by calling at her home (they have no telephone) but she was out. I eventually managed to contact Christopher's father at work and he was at the health centre in no time. Christopher was more than pleased to see him. He was seen by his doctor who advised treatment at the district general hospital; due to the nature of the injury he was taken to the hospital by his father. I wrote a letter to

Christopher's mother to inform her of what had happened and this was taken home by an older brother.

At the hospital Christopher had his hand X-rayed and the fingers were cleaned and dressed. In due course he returned to school. He still has some scarring on his fingers but has full use of them. His parents were very grateful for all that was done on Christopher's behalf and whilst he was at home kept me informed of his treatment and progress.

In accordance with local policy, accident report forms (personal injury) were made out in both cases, one copy being sent to the area education officer and the other retained in the medical room accident files. The accidents were also reported to the headmaster, the housemasters and tutors respectively.

A comparison of the job description of the occupational health nurse and the school nurse employed by the NHS shows considerable similarity except in respect of accidents and first-aid. However, the school nurse's occupational health responsibility may increase because it would seem sensible to reconsider and develop existing services, rather than institute new ones as the implementation of the 1974 Health and Safety at Work Act progresses. Area health authorities and local education authorities might consider examining the visiting occupational health services which have been set up and cooperatively financed by small factories in certain areas of the country. The visiting school nursing service could well be adapted along similar lines. Some schools have already set up safety committees and the doctor and nurse should certainly be members.

Prevention

This falls into the following main categories:

1. Well-constructed and maintained school buildings.
2. Safe use of transport to and from school.
3. Safety training as part of the subject curricula.
4. Regular practice for emergency situations.
5. Recording and investigation into accident aetiology as it affects school organization.

1. **Buildings** School building regulations aim to ensure that premises are safely constructed and give adequate protection for the children and staff. Ventilation, lighting, noise levels, planning, washing and toilet facilities are covered, and special considerations are given to buildings where handicapped children may be taught. The installation of equipment for gymnasiums, sports, practical work departments and laboratories, is strictly governed to prevent accident from faulty or unguarded items.

Both new and old buildings and all equipment needs to be well maintained and kept in good repair. Equipment and safety devices such as window catches need to be tested regularly and faulty objects should be prohibited from use until fully repaired and tested, or replaced. This is the responsibility of the head teacher, with support from the local education authority's building and works department. In residential schools items such as bedding and night clothing need to be of flame-proof materials.

2. Transport Road accidents are a major cause of death and injury among children. Therefore, it is not only necessary to see that safe transport is provided by the school or the parents but road safety teaching should have a high priority in the primary years. At present only about one-third of primary schools actively plan such programmes. The local authority road safety officer may be called in to advise on this and a number of road safety teaching schemes and proficiency tests are available. The Green Cross code is a particularly well known one. Accidents among teenagers starting to drive and ride mopeds or motorbikes are higher than for any other age-group[1] and schemes of training are being increasingly encouraged during the final school years in an effort to decrease the casualties.

3. Safety training The teaching of safe handling of equipment and prevention of accidents is the teacher's responsibility and should be automatically part of any lesson. Excellent guides to *Safety in Outdoor Pursuits, Science Laboratories, Practical Work Departments* and *Physical Education* have been issued by the DES and all staff should read them. The school health staff can draw attention to topics which need to be covered such as fireworks on Guy Fawkes' night or road safety.

4. Emergency practice There should be regular fire practice so that everyone in the school knows what action to take on finding a fire and how the building will be evacuated in a swift and orderly way. Fire-fighting equipment needs regular servicing, and fire doors must be used as intended.

5. Accident aetiology At present few schools keep good records of accidents and first-aid; consequently, there is no clear picture of environmental or individual factors affecting children, as for example, the length of time allocated for certain activities. Usually, only serious accidents are recorded and of these only a few warrant follow-up by an environmental officer.

Research in industry has tried to identify some of the social and physical causes of accidents. Factors in the individual may relate to previous experience of a job, age, sex, general health, sensorimotor ability, level of fatigue, general intelligence, emotional state and attitude towards the job. Contributory environmental factors may include lighting, noise, ventilation and temperature of the work place, and state and repair of equipment. The level of safety training and the use of safety devices also influence accident rates. All of these are equally applicable in the school.

First-Aid Responsibility

This is broadly the responsibility of everyone in the school—teachers, lay assistants and children alike. Unfortunately, first-aid is not routinely taught to children in school although some schools include it as an extra curricula activity when children join the Junior Red Cross or St John Ambulance Brigade. The local youth service could do a lot to assist in promoting this. Some teachers may also include it with safety in subjects where there is a high risk of certain accidents, for example, the swimming instructor may see that all children are taught the 'kiss of life' and not only those who are taking life-saving instruction.

Personnel with Major Responsibility

Generally every school has one or two designated first-aiders, often the head or one of the teachers in a small school, and possibly several teachers and lay helpers in a large school. First-aiders are generally responsible to the head teacher except in independent boarding schools where they are usually responsible to the sanitorium sister who keeps in regular contact, reviewing the records and dealing with serious complaints. Some maintained schools employ full-time school nurses to deal with first-aid. There is certainly a need for close working co-operation between the nurse and first-aider as it is here that the first indication of stress or problems arise, often in the shape of abdominal pains, or frequent headaches. First-aiders should have a recognized certificate issued by the St John Ambulance Brigade, St Andrew's Ambulance Association or the British Red Cross Society. These certificates have a limited validity of three years at the end of which the first-aider should attend another course or responsibility be passed to someone who has a current certificate. This ensures that practice is up to date and regularly revised.

First-aiders responsibilities

1. Attending to any minor injuries or complaints such as cuts and bruises, or headaches.
2. Keeping a daily record book with the names of the children and the nature of the complaint.
3. Seeing that first-aid boxes are kept fully equipped and accessible.
4. Being fully conversant with the procedures to adopt in case of accident or illness.
5. Identifying hazards in the school and instituting action in relation to these.
6. Knowing where gas and electricity main switches are sited in case of emergency.
7. Regularly up-dating their knowledge of first-aid.

1. *Minor first-aid* First-aid other than emergencies should be administered in either the medical room or a suitable area where there is a chair for the child to sit on, and running water for the first-aider to wash hands. A suitable bin for

soiled dressings should be at hand. Equipment should be confined to the first-aid box and not kept in desk drawers or lying about on open shelves. There also needs to be a policy on administration and use of patent medicines. A couch or chair-bed with blankets and pillow and a hot-water bottle should be available in case a child needs to lie down.

2. *Daily records* Records of minor first-aid are helpful if kept daily, particularly in large schools, in detecting children who are constantly complaining. These may also tie in with frequent brief absences from school. Complaints include headaches, abdominal pains, earaches, sore throats, hay-fever and minor skin complaints, and dysmennorhoea in adolescent girls. This information should be available to the doctor who will decide whether it indicates a more serious problem or some individual health education. For example, a sudden bout of fainting fits or hysteria may be the result of children starting to experiment with drugs of one kind or another. These also form part of the investigation into accident aetiology described on p. 172.

3. *First-aid boxes* These should be kept in strategic parts of the school and it is recommended that there should be one in every laboratory, practical work department, sports and physical recreation area. The school-bus should also be equipped and a suitable box needs to be kept for school journeys. There are many designs and types of boxes available, the best of which are designed and sold by the British Red Cross or recommended by the Industrial Health and Safety Centre. More specific guidance may soon be available from the Health and Safety Executive who are at present reviewing first-aid provision in work places. First-aid boxes should be accompanied by an instruction book to which additions may be made if there are children in the school suffering from complaints such as epilepsy, asthma or haemophilia which may require emergency treatment.

4. *Serious accidents* First-aid should be administered immediately and the child sent to hospital, escorted by the school matron or a member of the staff as appropriate. Information should be extracted from the teacher's medical information sheet and sent with the child. This should include:

1. The name and address of the child and where the parent or guardian may be contacted.
2. Family practitioner's name and address.
3. Immunization state (particularly tetanus in cases of sports-ground accidents).
4. Any allergies, illnesses or handicaps.
5. Date, time and brief details of the accident.

The head teacher will endeavour to inform the parents and will require an accident report either from the teacher concerned or the head will produce it himself. These are generally entered in a special book kept for the purpose and a copy is sent to the education authority. A copy of the report or a note of the accident should also be made in the medical record.

5. *Identifying hazards in the school* The importance of safe and well-maintained buildings has already been mentioned and responsibility for regular surveillance and checking of safety devices is usually best placed with the first-aider. The need for repairs and replacements should be brought to the attention of the head teacher and additional advice obtained from the school nurse or doctor.

6. *The site of switches for mains services* All main switches for gas, electricity and water need to be known by the first-aider and several responsible members of staff so that the source may be quickly turned off in the event of accident.

7. *Regularly up-dating knowledge of first-aid* Techniques change and newer more effective ways are found to deal with accidents; equally, practice which is throught to be good may be found lacking and fall into disrepute. Skills are only maintained if they are constantly practised and up-dated; consequently, first-aiders need to see that they attend re-training courses regularly. This applies equally to nurses as to lay first-aiders, although the general public and for some reason nurses themselves often feel they are exempt from this by virtue of a nursing qualification.

Particular problems Schools have particular responsibilities in relation to handicapped children and non-accidental injury.

Handicapped children First-aiders and teachers should be aware of any handicapped child in the school and the condition should be fully explained by the doctor or nurse with detailed instructions as to how to cope in an emergency. This is only fair to the teacher, the child and the other children in the class. An attack of epilepsy may be extremely frightening unless fully understood by the adults. Similarly, any drug treatment or change of drugs should be known so that any adverse effects may be noticed. Handicapped children are more likely to be accident-prone and arrangements for easy identification in case of accident are described on p. 114.

Non-accidental injury A great deal has been talked about non-accidental injury in the last few years and a lot of time has gone into training staff to be aware of the problem, to recognize it and to institute help for the child and the parents or guardian. This is by no means confined to very young children and first-aiders: play supervisors and teachers, particularly physical education teachers, are often the first to notice unusual or unexplained injuries; indeed, children suffering from this type of injury may suddenly refuse to undress for physical education. Teeth marks, burns or scratches on unlikely parts of the body and which do not tally with the child's explanation are all suspect. The local procedure for dealing with these suspicions should be followed and a copy of the procedure guide-lines needs to be in the school. In general the child should be seen by a doctor or dentist (in a case of teeth marks) as soon as possible. Delay will make it more difficult to be sure of the diagnosis as the marks will fade. If the nurse sees the child in the meantime, she should notice and record exact location of the marks, the size, severity, degree of inflammation, any infection and the state of healing.

REFERENCES

1. Ministry of Transport & Environment (1977) *Road Accidents—Great Britain 1975*. London: HMSO.

FURTHER READING

British Red Cross Society. *The ABC of First-aid*. London: Mills & Lacy. Ready reference and frequently included in the first-aid box.

British Red Cross Society (1975) *First-aid*, 4th impression. London: Mills & Lacy. The authorized manual.

British Red Cross Society. *First-aid questions and answers*. Wakefield, Yorkshire: E. P. Publishing.

Carter, J. (1974) *The Maltreated Child*. Hove, Sussex: Priory Press.

Consumer Association *Which* London: 14, Buckingham Street WC2. 01 839 1222. Gives information on the quality of consumer goods, including nightwear materials, etc., available from local library.

DES (1972) *Safety in Outdoor Pursuits*. London: HMSO, Safety Series.

DES (1973) *Safety in Physical Education* London: HMSO, Safety Series.

DES (1973) *Safety in Practical Departments*. London: HMSO, Safety Series.

DES (1973) *Safety in Science Laboratories*. London: HMSO, Safety Series.

CHILDREN'S BOOKS

Gydal, M. & Danielsson, T. (1976) *When Olly Went to Hospital*. Sevenoaks, Kent: Hodder and Stoughton. Olly goes into hospital for observation—illustrates hospital quite well. 5+ years.

Heseltine, M. (1973) *Bri's Accident*. London: MacMillan. Bri has an accident playing football in the street and attends the casualty for first-aid. 7+ years.

Pinkus, S. (1973) *Going into Hospital*. Hove, Sussex: Wayland. Covers wide area of hospital organization and procedure; should be discussed with an adult. 12+ years.

USEFUL ADDRESSES AND INFORMATION

British Red Cross Society
9 Grosvenor Crescent
London SW1
Tel: 01 235 5454

Sales and information on first-aid equipment and training courses for juniors.

British Safety Centre
62 Chancellors Road
London W6
Tel: 01 741 1231
   Provides training in safety, gives technical advice, produces posters and teaching materials, shows films and arranges lectures.

Health and Safety Executive
Baynards House
1 Chepstow Place
London W2 4TF
Tel: 01 229 3456
   Offer information on all aspects of the law and advice on specific queries. Publish a wide range of leaflets and booklets.

Industrial Health and Safety Centre
98 Horseferry Road
London SW1P 2D4
Tel: 01 828 9255
   Exhibition of industrial machinery with safety devices. Also first-aid boxes and special projects. Guided tours on request. Open 10 00 a.m. to 4 30 p.m.

NSPCC: National Advisory Centre for the Battered Child
Denver House
The Drive
Bounds Green Road
London N11
Tel: 01 361 1181
   Work includes teaching and advisory service on all aspects of non-accidental injury.

Royal Society for the Prevention of Accidents
Cannon House
The Priory
Queensway
Birmingham B4 6BS
Tel: 021 (Birmingham) 233 2461
   Deal with all aspects of accident information and prevention. Produce teaching materials and a quarterly magazine *Safety Education* specifically aimed at schools.

St Andrew's Association
48 Milton Street
Glasgow
Tel: 041 (Glasgow) 332 4031
   Training courses in first aid; also information.

St John Ambulance Brigade
1 Grosvenor Crescent
London SW1
Tel: 01 235 5231
   Training courses and information.

Discussion Topics

1. A child in the school is found to have lead poisoning. What action would you expect to be taken in the school?

2. You are a visiting school nurse in a city primary school. There is no road safety teaching undertaken in the school. How might you influence the school to start such teaching?

3. There are two epileptic children, an asthmatic and a diabetic attending ordinary school. What action would this lead you to take in relation to first-aid?

4. The first-aider's records show that large numbers of children from one particular class-room are constantly complaining of headaches. What might be the possible causes and what action would you take?

5. The swimming instructor asks you to look at a child with three symmetrical round scabs on his back. The child says he was scratched by the cat. How might you handle the situation?

6. You take up a post as a visiting school nurse and find that there is no trained first-aider in one of the schools. Discuss the sort of action which might alter the situation.

Conclusion

Chapter 11 dealt with the setting of aims and objectives and the importance of testing whether the teaching had been effective. The preface of this book stated my aims and objectives in producing this work as an instrument of equipping nurses to plan and organize their work in schools. I have no formal method of finding out whether I have added to the nurse's knowledge and understanding, and the assessment as to how she uses such information must be left to other members of the school team and the nursing officer in charge.

Self-testing is no bad thing and is something one can set up at any time throughout one's career. This can be particularly useful as an occasional exercise in school using actual histories and examining the success or failure of the actions taken and analysing the reasons so that good practice may be recognized and repeated and mistakes may be rectified. It is usually the function of the nursing officer to help the nurse in this and provide an objective view-point when case-loads are reviewed from time to time.

The following case history illustrates the kind of situation that might be analysed and the sort of questions that need to be asked and answered. (Although this case history is based on actual events, the names, ages and circumstances of the family have been altered to protect their interests.)

Case History	*Points for Discussion*
Mrs Brown aged 33 years	
Mr Brown aged 38 years	
James aged 9 years (illegitimate child)	
Gillian aged 7 years (in care of social services in another local authority)	
Caron aged 3 years (attending day nursery)	

Case History

At the beginning of 1972 this family arrived in London and lived in 'bed and breakfast' accommodation for seven weeks. The nature of any social work involvement there may have been is not known.

James did not attend school and no referral was made to the health visitor.

In April 1972 the family were rehoused and James started to attend the junior school. It was discovered that the family had previously lived in Wales and Liverpool. The addresses of previous schools were obtained and records were sent for but these were not forthcoming, and in May when James had his school entry medical his records were not available. His mother attended the medical.

Background History

Mrs Brown is a registered physically disabled person. She is very spastic and has great difficulty in walking and also has a bad speech impediment. Mr Brown manages to be employed in casual jobs from time to time but has long stretches of unemployment.

James was born before his mother's marriage and is the son of another man. Gillian has been in care since shortly after birth following a suspected battering and Caron attends the council day nursery because of the family history. Her place was obtained for her by a social worker in the social services department.

First Medical

James appeared physically fit but was reported by his teacher to be slow and demonstrating behaviour problems. Mrs Brown said that she was having marital difficulties and Mr Brown did not get on at all well with James.

Following medical examination it was decided that in view of the family history the child should be seen at school medicals every two months and

Points for Discussion

Should this family have been notified to the health visitor and what action might be taken to prevent this omission in the future?

What could be done to improve movement of school records?

What special surveillance might be considered in view of this history?

First Medical

that teachers, social workers, the school nurse and doctor should observe him closely for any sign of bruising and ill-treatment. It was decided that the social worker already dealing with the family should be asked to make a home visit and submit a written report on the family situation.

Second Medical

James was seen again after two months. No verbal or written report had been received from the social worker. No signs of ill-treatment had been observed but his behaviour was reported to have deteriorated even more. He was accompanied by his father who told the school nurse that he was having marital difficulties but could not wait to see the doctor and left before James was seen. Because of his behaviour problems the school doctor asked for James to be seen by the educational psychologist. He was physically fit but his general appearance and clothing were dirty and unkempt. The voluntary worker contacted the education welfare officer who visited the family and a grant for clothing was obtained.

The family had now moved to another address and consequently have a new social worker from the social services department. The voluntary worker also visited and established a good relationship with the family.

Summer Holiday

During the six-week summer holiday no visits were made.

September 1972

Mrs Brown was seen by the head teacher who explained that James was to be seen by the educational psychologist as she thought that James was slow in learning and disorderly in class. Mrs Brown wondered if this was the result of a severe accident he had when aged three years. There was no way of checking this information as all records were still unavailable.

Points for Discussion

Might these problems have been dealt with in alternative ways?

Was this wise? What could have been done during the holiday?

October 1972

The school called a case conference which was attended by the education welfare officer, the voluntary worker, the school nurse and doctor, and the head teacher. Unfortunately, the social worker from the social services department was unable to attend and there was no report available. It was felt at this stage that James could no longer be contained within the school. An appointment with the educational psychologist could not be obtained for some considerable time. James was referred to the assessment clinic at the district general hospital. The voluntary worker took James and his mother to the hospital weekly for some weeks and the child psychologist recommended that James should attend a day school for the maladjusted as soon as a vacancy became available, and in the meantime he should be given some remedial teaching.

To date, no previous educational, health or social services records have been available.

Points for Discussion

How do you think the handling of this situation could be improved?

Index

Index